1001 little
SKINCARE
MIRACLES

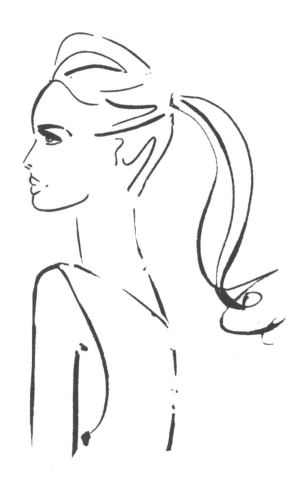

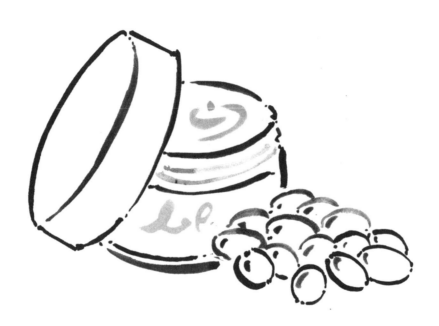

1001 little SKINCARE MIRACLES

Esme Floyd

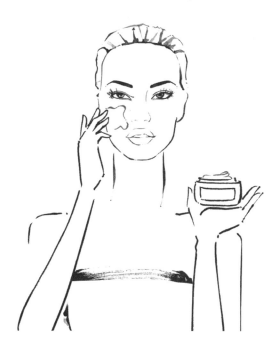

CARLTON
BOOKS

THIS IS A CARLTON BOOK

Text and design copyright © 2013
Carlton Books Limited
Illustrations by Kerri Hess

This edition published by
Carlton Books Limited 2013
20 Mortimer Street
London W1T 3JW

A CIP catalogue record for this book is available from the
British Library.

ISBN: 978-1-78097-299-2

Printed and bound in China

This book reports information and opinions which may be
of general interest to the reader. Neither the author nor the
publisher can accept responsibility for any accident, injury
or damage that results from using the ideas, information
or advice offered in this book.

The advice in this book is general in nature, not specific
to individuals or their particular circumstances. Any plant
substance, whether used as a medicine or a food, externally
or internally, can cause an allergic reaction in some people.
Do not try self-diagnosis or attempt self-treatment for
serious or long-term problems without consulting a medical
professional or qualified practitioner. Do not use essential
oils or herbal preparations without prior consultation with
a medical professional if you are pregnant, taking any form
of medication or if you suffer from sensitive skin. Always
seek medical advice if symptoms persist.

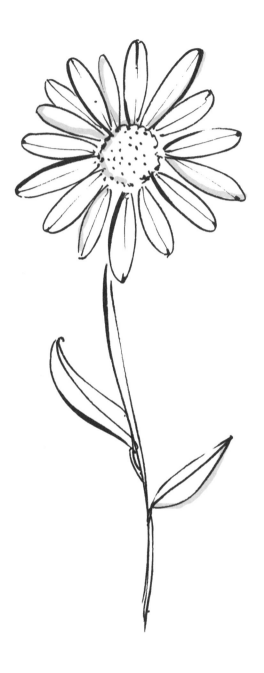

CONTENTS

INTRODUCTION

Did you know that your skin isn't just a cover for your body? It's actually the largest organ. The skincare industry is a multibillion dollar business, and it's growing bigger every day, with almost a quarter of all global beauty sales dedicated to skincare products. But with hundreds of new products, ingredients and techniques flooding the market every month, and amidst all those claims about scientific ingredients, cosmeceuticals and miracle cures, just how are real women – and men – supposed to find their own path to glowing, gorgeous skin?

This book is your unique everyday, practical guide through this highly technical world, revealing the latest tips and advice to help you create and maintain a flawless complexion from head to toe. From the latest miracle ingredients and dietary tips to techniques and advice for all types of skin, from medical advice to help solve skin problems to tips on wrinkles, cellulite and sailing through the seasons, this beauty insider's guide will tell you everything you need to know to keep your skin healthy and happy, whatever your age or budget.

roll of honour

Everyone's skin is different, and varying lifestyles, health requirements, environments, age and emotional states mean our skin needs different things to keep it in tip-top condition, but the best advice is the simplest. Your skin is an organ and there's no doubt it's what you put *into* your body – in terms of diet, activity, supplements and quality of sleep – rather than what you put on it that holds the majority of the keys to skin health.

But there are some global products and brands whose names crop up over and over again when it comes to the gold standards of skincare, and although this book isn't about products – it's about simple decisions and actions you can take to help your skin look and feel its best – we couldn't let go the opportunity to say a big congratulations to some of our favourite simply fantastic skincare products ... enjoy!

SUPERSTAR: EVE LOM

For many years, Eve Lom has been the top choice of skincare professionals, celebrities and editors alike. With extracts of plants and herbs and a unique hot cloth/massage application and removal, it cleans, tones, exfoliates and nourishes the skin in one go. Simply invest in a pot of cleanser, or get a total Eve Lom overhaul with cleanser, morning time cleanser, TLC cream, eye cream and serum. See www.evelom.com.

BRAND SUPERSTAR ... BIO-OIL

Beloved of dry skin everywhere, this simple formulation of PurCellin Oil mixed with plant extracts has been shown to help skin repair itself. It's a favourite with people all over the globe. Pregnant women use it to avoid stretch marks, it helps with scar reduction, and is also used for deep moisturizing dry skin and treating feet, elbows and even lips. The appeal is simple – one oil, one product, many uses. A must for everyone's beauty shelf! See www.bio-oil.com.

BRAND SUPERSTAR ... TRILOGY

Trilogy has a reputation for high-class, maximum effect skincare with a minimal effect on the environment. Their range covers face and bodycare as well as specialist products, but the shining star is Organic Rosehip Oil, because rosehips have the highest levels of Vitamin A (Retinol) of pretty much anything alive, and a whole range of other antioxidant vitamins too, and this oil is extracted from the seeds of certified organic wild-grown rosehips to help give dull, tired or damaged skin back its bounce and glow. See www.trilogyproducts.com.

BRAND SUPERSTAR ... PHILIPS

Lots of different companies make hair removal products, but Philips has consistently shown itself to be ahead of the game. Whether it's a smooth shave from razors or Ladyshave, long-term hair removal with epilators (our favourite is the Satin Perfect Wet and Dry) or the new Lumea laser removal system, they've got it right. And watch this space for skincare, too, as they launch the at-home RéAura Laser Skin Rejuvenation tool, based on Fraxel laser technology. See www.philips.co.uk.

BRAND SUPERSTAR ... OBAGI

Across the globe, Obagi is *the* go-to brand for those with skin problems such as acne scarring, sun damage or dry, dehydrated and ageing skin. The powerful but non-abrasive formulations are available worldwide on prescription from medical professionals, so ask your doctor or dermatologist for advice. See www.obagi.com.

PRODUCT SUPERSTARS

Special mentions also must go to Korres for their fabulous body butters, Aromatherapy Associates for harnessing the power of essential oils so beautifully, Naked Skincare for making paraben-free products affordable, Oskia for their top-of-the-class MSM supplement (and a rather wonderful papaya face peel as well), Burt's Bees for the best lip balm, Ren Skincare for their Moroccan Rose Otto range and Clarins for their Blue Orchid Face Treatment Oil, because when something smells *that* good, the fact that it works a treat to rehydrate dry skin is an added bonus!

Top ten little skincare miracles

We hope you have fun reading about our miracles – here's a taster of 10 of the author's very own favourites ...

37

WIPE YOUR PHONE
(See Lifestyle Tips, page 19)

42

MEASURE YOUR STRESS
(See Lifestyle Tips, page 20)

98

SLEEP EASY
(See Get Your Beauty Sleep, page 31)

352

GIVE NATURE A HAND
(See Arms and Legs, page 85)

442

GO EASY ON THE SHIMMER
(See Regular and Tinted
Moisturizers, page 102)

661

GET A B-GRADE
(See Anti-ageing Nutrition, page 149)

936

SAY NO TO CHOCOLATE
(See Cold Sores, page 208)

945

DO A CLEOPATRA
(See Eczema, page 210)

966

GET DEAD AHEAD
(See Psoriasis, page 215)

986

KNOW YOUR ALPHABET
(See Freckles, Moles
& Birthmarks, page 219)

HEALTH & NUTRITION

understanding your skin type

1 IDENTIFY YOUR SKIN TYPE

In order to choose the right skincare products, you need to know your skin type. Dry skin usually has an uneven skin tone, visible capillaries (veins) and flakiness, while oily skin is more prone to visible pores, breakouts and areas of pigmentation. Despite its name, normal skin is the rarest skin type. It is clear, smooth, soft and supple, with even tone, texture and pigment, few or no blemishes, good levels of hydration and no sensitive areas.

2 DON'T BE A DRY BABY

Dry skin is not the same as dehydrated skin, although a lack of moisture can make the symptoms worse. Quick to tighten, flake and the first type of skin on which fine lines appear, dry skin needs immediate action. Study your diet and lifestyle choices for the answers. Medication, alcohol, hormonal changes and poor nutrition can all be causes.

3 GET IN THE T-ZONE

If you have combination skin, treat the different areas of your face independently – exfoliate the T-zone more regularly than cheeks, and when moisturizing concentrate on cheeks and neck, leaving only a light layer or none at all if not required on the T-zone.

4 SPLIT PERSONALITY

You know the skin on your face and body are different, so you use different products on them, right? Do the same if you have different skin on different areas of your face and body – what's right for cheeks, for instance, might not be right for nose and chin.

5 RISE AND SHINE

If your skin shines, especially on the T-zone down the middle of your face, you have at least some areas of oily skin, and the time of day it starts shining after your morning regime tells you how oily it is – by mid-morning it's very oily, by teatime less so. The benefits of oily skin are that wrinkles are slow to appear, but regular deep cleansing is a must to avoid open, shiny pores.

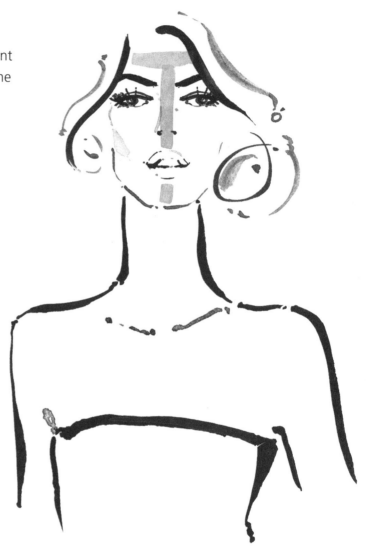

6 CLEANSE DEEPLY

For oily skin, and oily areas of combination skin, make sure you get a really good level of cleansing – deep cleansing will help lower the activity of oil-generating sebaceous glands under the skin, which in turn reduces the likelihood of blackheads and spots.

7 DON'T BE HARSH

If your skin is prone to dryness and sometimes feels very tight, itchy or sore, or if it becomes easily inflamed and irritated, you have sensitive skin. It's extremely important to reduce the use of harsh products (containing soap or alcohol) and protect your skin against external stressors.

8 DO A WIPE TEST

To determine your skin type, just after you wake up in the morning wipe your face with a clean facial tissue. If the tissue is left clean with no traces of oil and feels fine after wiping, you have normal skin; if the tissue is clean but your face feels tight, it's dry. Spots of facial oil will reveal oily areas, and may reveal your skin is oily or combination (where cheeks are dry but the forehead, nose and chin are oily).

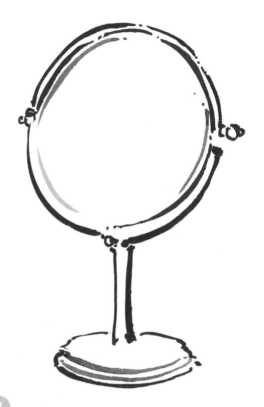

9 MAGNIFY CHANGES

The texture of skin alters frequently depending on environmental factors like pollution and weather so you should change your skin products accordingly. To check up on the current state of your skin, hold a magnifying mirror up close to your cleansed face in bright daylight and look for clues like patches of dryness, oiliness or breakouts.

10 DON'T BE A CHEEKY CHAPPY

If your cheeks are red with broken capillaries and skin often feels tight, flushed or blushing, don't automatically assume you have Rosacea, a chronic inflammatory skin condition causing redness but also blemishes and lumps under the skin's surface. There is also a skin type known as "couperose" skin, which is red-cheeked and sensitive, especially on cheeks.

11 GO GENTLY

Couperose skin and rosacea can seem similar, but the treatments are different. Couperose skin will benefit from a simple, uncomplicated routine with gentle, scent-free products. Also, avoid using water that is too hot or cold, which may cause further redness, and any products containing too many active ingredients like botanicals or cosmeceuticals.

12 NORMAL WISDOM

If you have normal skin, make sure you choose a light moisturizer, especially one that is formulated as a lotion or gel. Too-rich moisturizers can trigger spots and blemishes in the oilier areas by blocking pores.

13 GO EASY ON YOUR CHEEKS

Sensitive skin is usually dry with fine pores and a tendency to redness, especially on the cheeks. It may react by reddening and feeling tight and sore in sunlight, wind, heat and cold or changes in humidity. Avoid using too many products as these could actually make skin more sensitive by overloading it.

14 DON'T BE A FLAKE

If your skin flakes or feels tight, especially on cheeks, forehead and the sides of your nose, you probably have dry skin. These symptoms are caused by a lack of sebum (skin oil), so choose products that protect against dehydration and help reduce skin damage.

15 TAKE THE BRIEF

If you suffer from dry skin, try not to spend too long in the bath or shower, and avoid over-cleansing your face. The constant wetting and drying serves to dehydrate your skin even more. Aim to reduce your time under water to five minutes a day if your skin is really dry and use soap every other day instead of daily, or apply a soft, soap free cleanser instead.

lifestyle tips

16 SEEK ADVICE

If you have any sort of skin problem that doesn't seem normal or your skin has changed a lot recently, ask for a referral to a dermatologist, or seek one privately. Look for the governing body for dermatologists in your area to ensure you are choosing someone reputable and check credentials carefully. Don't be afraid to ask what the letters after their name mean – any real expert will be only too glad to explain.

17 KEEP ON DRINKING

The number one tip for better skin, whatever your type, is to make sure you drink enough water. This is particularly important for dry skin, which is more prone to dehydration than other types. Drinking at least six glasses of water a day helps to suppress appetite, metabolize fat, and keep your body and skin fully hydrated and younger-looking. Fizzy drinks, herbal teas and fruit juice will not provide the same benefits as plain water.

18 STOP SMOKING

Smoking tobacco changes the skin's DNA repair process, which in turn leads to the breakdown of collagen and elastin fibres, resulting in premature lines and wrinkles. It also starves the skin of oxygen and essential nutrients, and severely dehydrates it, all of which causes premature ageing.

18 BEST OF THREE

When it comes to skincare, there's a three-minute rule – three minutes is the time it takes after showering, bathing or washing for skin to start to dehydrate. Make sure you apply your products (preferably to slightly damp skin) quickly to help lock in moisture and achieve the maximum hydrating effects.

20 LAYER YOUR CREAMS

It's a myth that the oilier and greasier the cream, the more it hydrates. Instead of thickening the layers of cream, add a light serum layer underneath to feed rather than choke skin.

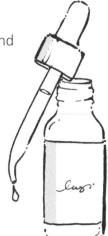

21 PARE DOWN YOUR BEAUTY BAG

It's all too tempting to accumulate a whole range of skincare products, but simple is usually best. Try to stick to one brand at a time as the products are designed to work in harmony, but keep it simple. A cleanser, day cream, night cream, body cream and hand/foot cream should be enough, and if you want to go a bit larger you could choose an eye cream and serum plus a face mask for weekly use.

22 SWEAT IT OUT

Nothing clears skin like a good sweat (as long as you cleanse and moisturize properly afterwards). Aim to do enough physical exercise to sweat at least five times a week for a minimum of 10 to 15 minutes to help detoxify and boost radiance.

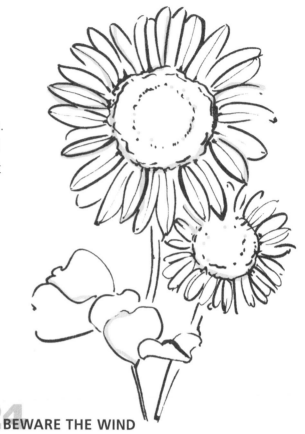

23 LOVE YOUR GLOVES

Gloves are great for protecting hands in the winter to prevent them from drying and chapping, and light cotton or muslin gloves can also protect skin from sun damage during the summer. Wear them as often as you can during the day to help keep skin moist and supple.

24 BEWARE THE WIND

Rain and wind can really play havoc with your skin, especially if it's prone to dryness. A moisturizer with natural oils is a good choice because it helps nourish the skin. Look for products with almond, sunflower and jojoba oils, which are all high in substances to help skin rejuvenate.

25 BREAK THE BOUNDARIES

For the purposes of using different creams and skincare products, your boundaries should look like this: 1. Face, neck and décolleté, 2. Rest of body, 3. Hands. If you suffer with dry skin on your feet, treat them like your hands, otherwise they go in with the rest of the body. Don't be tempted to use body cream on your neck and décolleté – face creams are a much better choice.

26 WAIT A MONTH

Even though it's what most marketing campaigns imply, don't expect overnight changes when you alter your skincare regime. If you're using a new cream or product, allow at least two weeks, preferably a month (or 10–12 weeks for anti-ageing products) before you make a decision about whether to continue using it. Your skin takes 28 days to totally regenerate, so as long as new products don't cause adverse reactions keep on using them for a while before you judge them.

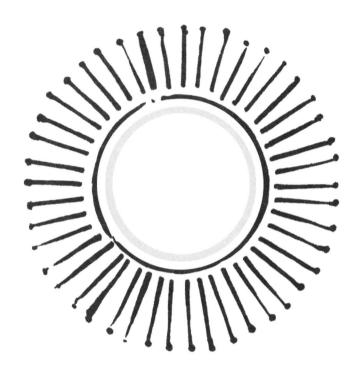

27 SOAK UP SOME EARLY RAYS

A great way to give your skin a dose of vitamin D-boosting sunshine without exposing it to the harmful rays of the midday sun is to expose it to the early morning or late evening sun, which has all the benefits but far fewer of the damaging effects. Exercise out in the open or simply sit and meditate for 15 minutes.

28 LISTEN TO YOUR BODY

If you've been ill, under the weather or on medication, look for changes in your skin type as you recover and adjust your skincare routine accordingly. Because your skin is an organ, illness affects it just like your other organs, and it might need a little extra TLC to get back to normal.

29 GO SEASONAL

Not everyone can afford a facial every four to six weeks as experts recommend, but if you can make it at the beginning of every season, your skin will thank you. As the seasons change, your skin changes too, and starting off the new season with a professional skin workout helps keep it looking tip-top.

30 BREAK BAD HABITS

Any repetitive movement such as chewing gum, frowning or sucking on a cigarette will lead to fine lines. Over time, micro-tears appear in the skin, resulting in collagen-damaging inflammation. Smoking causes you to squint and pucker, exaggerating wrinkles around the eyes and mouth.

31 DRY DAYS

One of the effects of alcohol is to cause small blood vessels in the skin to widen, allowing more blood flow into the skin's surface layers. This causes redness, which, if it happens regularly, can be permanent and leads to thread veins in the cheeks and nose. Many people assume alcohol's most damaging effect on the skin is dehydration and this can be offset by drinking lots of water, but don't forget alcohol is a powerful inflammatory agent, which can lead to many more skin problems than simple dryness. Moderation is key, so let your skin bounce back with at least three dry days a week.

32 AND BREATHE ...

Nothing has the power to damage the skin like stress; it's fine in the short term but long term, it can cause inflammatory responses, premature ageing and all sorts of other problems. Stress causes hormonal changes in the body that affect all the organs and show up most clearly on the skin, so make sure you incorporate some relaxation into your daily routine.

33 TURN IT DOWN

A hot, steamy bath or shower might seem like the best choice for relaxation, but it's not always best for your skin as it can cause drying and redness. For best results, keep the temperature warm but not hot, and if you want steam, set the kettle to boil then place a bowl of the hot water in the bathroom.

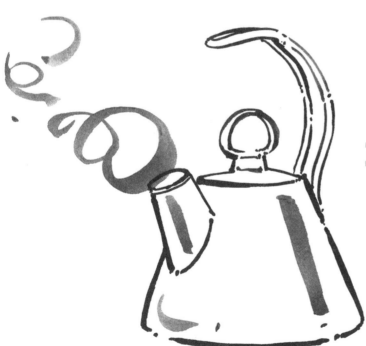

34 DON'T BE PLASTIC FANTASTIC

Some people believe that exposure of fatty foods to chemicals found in plastics can lead to an increase of hormones in the diet as the fats absorb some of the compounds – use paper, cardboard and glass instead of plastic bags and clingfilm (plastic wrap).

35 HOW LOW CAN YOU GO?

Low GI foods, which help regulate the body's sugar and insulin levels, can help your skin look better by reducing the inflammatory response and preventing overactive oil gland activity. Choose whole grains, vegetables and beans over white bread, rice, potatoes and sugar.

36 HAIR FIRST

If you're applying hair products, try to do so before you cleanse your face and apply your facial products, otherwise the hair products can interfere and even cause skin reactions such as oiliness and breakouts. Always do your hair first then your face to ensure the only products on your face are the ones you choose to apply!

37 WIPE YOUR PHONE

Several studies have shown that cell phones – which are held up close to, or touching the skin for many minutes or hours a day, not to mention all that action from fingers – can be real hotbeds for germs and bacteria. Wipe your phone daily with a cleansing or sanitizing wipe to keep it clean.

38 DON'T CHOKE ON SMOKE

Even if you don't smoke yourself, you'll no doubt be aware of the negative effects of second-hand smoke from passive smoking, and nowhere are these stronger than on the skin. Wherever possible, avoid being in smoky places and if friends or family smoke, ask them not to do so around you.

39 EXPERT ADVICE

Instead of being taken in by shiny packaging and clever marketing campaigns, ask an expert what products would work best for your skin. Even with the cost of a consultation, you'll probably save yourself money in the long run through making informed choices.

40 GET ACTIVE

It's amazing when you actually get down to reading the labels of products, how similar most generic brands are in terms of ingredients to their far more expensive designer cousins. Unless it's a patented formula or a particular mix of ingredients, it's likely that most skin creams contain roughly the same elements. Look at the amount of active ingredients to make your choice.

41 HEAL OVERNIGHT

As you sleep at night "stress" hormones such as cortisol and epinephrine (adrenalin) reduce and your body produces growth hormone (also nicknamed "the youth hormone") and melatonin, which help reduce inflammation and promote repair, but it's not until you enter your deep sleep stage that this change happens. Aim to get a good blast of uninterrupted sleep each night.

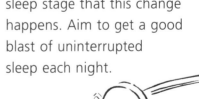

42 MEASURE YOUR STRESS

To get a measure of just how much pollution you expose your skin to, take a square of white fabric, such as silk, cotton or muslin, and carry it around with you all day so that it is exposed to everything your skin is exposed to (tie it to the outside of your handbag, or wear it as a scarf or headscarf). At the end of the day, take a peek and see just how much invisible dirt and grease has accumulated on your skin. You'll never skip cleansing again!

diet & nutrition

43 LOOK GREAT WITH GRAPES

Resveratrol, a polyphenol found in red grapes and an antioxidant and anti-cancer agent, helps mop up the damage caused by sun and pollution exposure, helping skin to heal itself following damage. In addition to eating grapes, look for vinotherapy salon treatments and products that claim to harvest this ingredient.

44 C CLEARLY

One of the key vitamins for skincare is vitamin C – this is because it's essential for the formation of collage, the "glue" structures that hold skin together and keep it looking firm. Aim for five to eight portions of fruit and vegetables a day (ideally more vegetables than fruit).

45 LIGHTEN UP

If you have dark circles under your eyes or bloating, this could be a result of inflammation in your skin, which is exacerbated by stress, sugar and processed foods. Eat lots of healthy fresh vegetables and fruit for a few days to flush away the swelling.

46 GET FISHY

There's no point investing in expensive creams and lotions if you don't help your skin from the inside as well. One of the best ways to do this is to make sure you have a diet rich in fish, which contains oils to help keep skin supple and reduce wrinkles. If you don't like the taste of fish, take fish oil supplements instead.

47 BE A PROTEIN PRO

A lack of protein can adversely affect the skin because protein cannot be stored in the body and therefore if your diet doesn't contain enough protein – from lean meat, fish, beans and pulses – the body must rely on its own resources, which are often the skin's support structures. If this continues, it can accentuate the ageing process.

48 FEED YOUR SKIN

Your skin is the last of your body's organs to receive the vitamins, minerals and nutrients you take in from food and supplements so if you don't get enough, your skin is first to suffer. That's why it's important to make sure your diet has the right level of vitamins and minerals to keep all your body's organs functioning optimally.

49 CUT THE FLAX

Flax seeds are a great source of omega-3 fatty acids, which help the skin regenerate and repair itself. To get your omega-3 fix, sprinkle a dessertspoon of flax onto breakfast cereals, or into yogurt.

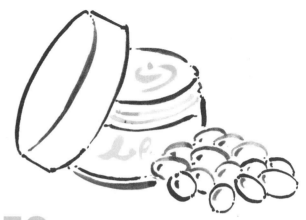

50 GO NUTS FOR VITAMIN E

Eating nuts such as walnuts and hazelnuts can help supply your skin with essential vitamin E, which improves skin tone and helps keep skin looking healthy and glowing. Sprinkle a few nuts onto breakfast cereal, yogurt or a salad to keep your E-levels topped up.

51 A-GRADE SALADS

A couple of times a week, give your body a vitamin A boost with an A-grade salad of orangey vegetables such as carrots, squash, sweet potatoes and tomatoes with broccoli and kale (or other green leafy vegetables). This is especially good if you have rough, dry skin, which can be caused by low vitamin A.

52 DEEP PURPLE

Anthocyanidins – often responsible for giving foods a dark red or purplish colour – are one of the body's best protections against damage, and unlike vitamin C (which works best in the watery parts of the body) and vitamin E (best in fatty areas), they work throughout the body. Black grapes, blueberries, cranberries and pine bark (pycnogenol) are all rich sources.

53 OIL IT UP

If you have dry skin, include lots of natural oils in your diet to help boost sebum production. Fish oils, eggs, olive oil, flaxseed oil and avocado are all good, healthy choices, and butter is good, if used sparingly.

54 SAY NO TO SUGAR

Refined sugar and white flour can help create skin problems, lead to premature ageing and increase wrinkles by taking its toll on all the body's systems. Avoid processed foods and added sugar, and try to restrict white floury products to every other day at most.

55 CUT DOWN ON DAIRY

If you find your skin is prone to blackheads, oiliness and breakouts, it might be worth reducing your milk and dairy intake, as there is some anecdotal evidence that the hormones contained in dairy products can lead to breakouts. Although not scientifically sound, it's worth a try if you're suffering spotty skin.

56 MAKE IT A MACKEREL

There's a lot of information about salmon and omega oils, but there are plenty of other – cheaper – fish, which are an excellent source of oils for your skin. If your tastebuds (or your wallet) don't like salmon, try sardines, mackerel and anchovies (fresh, not salted) instead.

57 SAY OOH FOR OMEGA

Omega-3 oils have been shown to control the production of leukotriene B4, which can cause acne and skin inflammation. To up your levels of omega 3, take a supplement daily or add the usual omega suspects to your diet every day – walnuts, avocados, flaxseed oil and oily fish are all great choices.

58 GET SEEDY

Seeds and seafood are excellent skin choices because they are high in zinc, which helps the body make its two most powerful antioxidant enzymes. Selenium and manganese are also needed, but they are usually present in the same foods as zinc.

59 CHOOSE WATERMELON

Watermelon is one of the best foods for a quick vitamin boost – the flesh is high in vitamin C and beta-carotene (which the body uses to make vitamin A), and the seeds are high in vitamin E, selenium and zinc. Blend up the flesh and seeds to make sure you receive all the benefits.

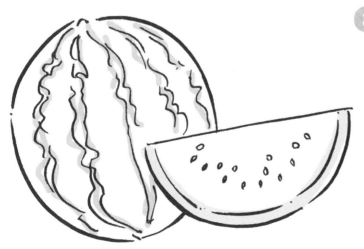

60 GO ORANGE

Orange and red foods are ideal ingredients for healthy skin because they contain high levels of beta-carotene, which is essential for the skin to produce the vitamins it needs to help protect it from antioxidant and UV damage. Sweet potatoes, peppers, carrots and squash are all great choices.

61 GET THE BALANCE RIGHT

Most modern diets contain far too much sodium (from salt) and not enough magnesium and potassium (found in fresh fruit and vegetables). Opt for low sodium sea salt if you use it in cooking, avoid processed foods and cured meats and eat lots of fresh vegetables.

62 ENJOY REGULAR PORTIONS

Studies have shown that vitamins A, C and E can actually help to prevent the skin from being as damaged by UV rays as it would without these vitamins, which is perhaps why diets in sunny climates always seem to contain so much fresh fruit and vegetables, the key dietary source. Eat regular portions throughout the day to keep levels topped up.

63 JOIN THE Q

Another vital antioxidant is Coenzyme-Q10, also known as Co-Q10. Because we can make it in our own bodies, it's not classed as a vitamin but it's a great way to make sure the body has antioxidant power. You'll find it in meat and fish (particularly sardines), green vegetables, soy and wheatgerm.

64 GO ORGANIC

One of the best ways to ensure that you're not taking in damaging toxins with your diet is to choose organic or free-range additive-free foods, which you know won't have been unnecessarily exposed to pollutants such as pesticides, antibiotics or fertilizers. Make sure, too, that you wash your fruit and vegetables before eating. Not only does washing remove unpalatable dirt or earth, it also ensures your fresh foods don't contain residues of chemicals from the growing, picking, packing or transportation process that they've undergone before reaching your plate.

vitamins & minerals

65 GET SOME ZZS

If there's one mineral you should make sure you include in your diet for healthy, smooth skin, it's zinc. Essential for helping the skin to regulate moisture and oil levels – and therefore prevent breakouts – and strengthen it from the inside out, you'll find zinc in most multivitamins, green vegetables and seafood.

66 REACH FOR ROSEMARY

Rosemary is a great source of vitamin E, and rosemary extract or rosemary oil extract is often used to add to natural supplements or fish oils to inject a dose of the antioxidant vitamin. Look out for it if you need an extra skin boost.

67 SEEK OUT SELENIUM

Fish, red meat, chicken, grains and eggs all contain selenium, an antioxidant that works with vitamin E against pollutants to combat skin ageing and cancer. Healthy sources include oil-rich nuts, seeds and avocados.

68 BE ALERT TO BETA-CAROTENE

Beta-carotene, a powerful natural anti-ageing antioxidant, is a pigment in yellow and red fresh foods that the body converts to vitamin A to generate new cells. You'll find it in apricots, peaches, nectarines, sweet potatoes, carrots and leafy greens.

68 MIX UP SOME MSM

MSM is the most readily absorbed version of sulphur, which has long been understood to be beneficial for bones, joints, nails, hair and skin in order for them to grow and function optimally. The best version on the market is the Canadian OptiMSM, which is the only form to go through a four-stage distillation process for optimal purity (available from Oskia Skincare).

70 GET A GA

Native Americans have long used the bark and resin from larch trees to help skin renewal, tighten skin, reduce wrinkles and prevent dehydration. In natural beauty products, look for the modern version as GA (galactoarabinan) to harness its benefits.

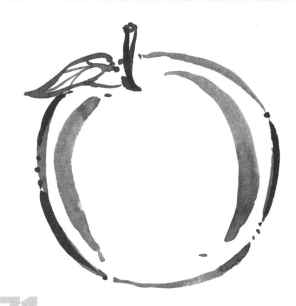

71 BE AN A-STUDENT

The recommended daily allowance of vitamin A is around 3,000 IU, but be careful not to have too much more than that, especially if you are breastfeeding or pregnant or you suffer from a weakened immune system. It also appears on labels as acetate. You may well not see vitamin A on the label of your supplements, but you might spot beta-carotene instead – the raw material the body needs to make its own vitamin A. Try not to take more than 15,000 IU beta-carotene a day – instead load up with fresh fruit and vegetables.

72 D FOR DELIGHT

If you're over 45, taking vitamin D and folic acid (B vitamin complex) daily is a great choice because it helps the skin repair itself and therefore reduces wrinkles. Look for 400ug folic acid and a minimum of 400IU vitamin D, as well as seeking out daylight for at least 20 minutes a day.

supplements

73 BE A CHEMIST

A sure-fire way to ensure you're not being fobbed off with a low-quality oil is to check that whatever you buy is labelled pharmaceutical grade, with a certificate of analysis and third party tested. That way, you can be sure you're choosing well.

74 GO ONLINE

There is an international website for an organization called IFOS, which is the International Fish Oil Standards, that many fish oils are signed up to for third party testing. Check this, or other independent consumer websites, to see how different supplements compare.

75 DON'T SIN WITH SYNTHETICS

It is possible to make synthetic versions of vitamin C and E in a laboratory, but these are not natural versions and there are differences in functions, absorption and breakdown in the body. Instead look for natural d-tocopherol and calcium ascorbate.

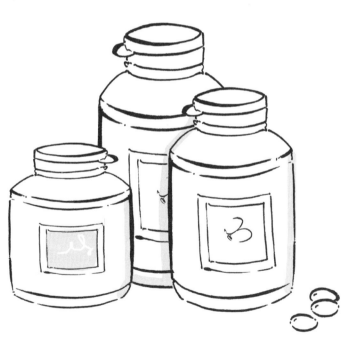

76 PRICE ISN'T EVERYTHING

Don't assume that the most expensive supplement is necessarily the best – some vitamin companies price their products highly simply because they spend so much on their advertising costs. However, the lower-cost supplements might contain synthetic ingredients or high levels of fillers to bulk up products. Rather than basing your decisions purely on money, study the labels carefully to decide which supplements you should buy.

77 KEEP IT SIMPLE

Instead of taking several pills, choose a supplement that contains all the ingredients you need in one pill – there are so many different supplements on the market that it shouldn't be hard to find one that fits your particular needs. Avoid supplements that contain more filler and added ingredients than pure vitamin, and steer clear of brands with large amounts of sugar, starch, iron, wheat, dairy, salt, cellulose, artificial colours and flavourings and artificial preservatives.

78 BUY REGULARLY

Because fish oils are natural, even though they've been purified they do degrade over time. Keep yours refrigerated and try to buy a smaller bottle so you're not keeping it for more than a few months before you replace with a fresh source. Always choose a fish oil supplement that is completely natural, rather than synthetic. The natural triglyceride form is the best way to help your body derive the most benefit from fish oils, as it's evolved over many thousands of years.

79 LOOK AT THE LABEL

A popular trick for disguising low-quality, low-grade fish oils in supplements is to simply state they are "fish oil" without listing the separate amounts or ratios for the different omega-3 fatty acids, DHA, EPA and DPA, or the fish source. The sum of these three fatty acids should add up to at least 100 mg of the total omega-3 amount; if there's a big gap, the supplement is probably full of synthetic oils, which are not so potent.

80 DON'T BELIEVE THE HYPE

When it comes to buying a supplement, there are some phrases that you should take with a pinch of salt. There is no specific meaning for words like "high potency", "super", "total" or "natural", which means in theory anyone could use them on a label. For the real low-down, look at specific amounts and the manufacturing process.

81 GO ALGAL

If you are worried about eating fish oil, are vegetarian or allergic to fish, try algae oil instead. It has many of the same health benefits but is derived from marine algae.

82 RELATE TO CHELATED

Chelated minerals are often recommended, as their claw-like shape enables them to be better absorbed into the body because they don't bind so readily to food, which blocks the absorption process. Chelated calcium, for instance, is around 10 per cent more easily absorbed than non-chelated, but it costs a whopping three to five times more, so it's up to you to decide if it's worth the extra.

detoxing through diet

83 TAKE CARE WITH CALCIUM

Taking an antioxidant vitamin supplement is a great way to help your body detox and they are usually better if taken with meals. Try to avoid taking anything containing calcium at the same time, though, as the mineral can block vitamin absorption – leave your calcium supplement until between meals, and avoid dairy products when you pop your pill.

84 TAKE A PILL

If you're doing a detox, boost your body's natural detox capabilities with supplements. Specialist detox supplements are the ideal choice for short-term use and psyllium husks (an excellent source of dietary fibre) can help remove toxins. Aim to include one portion of detox foods like spirulina or alfalfa sprouts per day in your diet to boost your intake of nutrients that can help the detoxification process.

85 PACK A PINEAPPLE PUNCH

Pineapple contains a natural substance called bromelain that acts as a natural anti-inflammatory in the joints and skin. Try drinking a glass of fresh pineapple juice (with no added sugar) in the morning and eat some fresh pineapple in the evening throughout your detox.

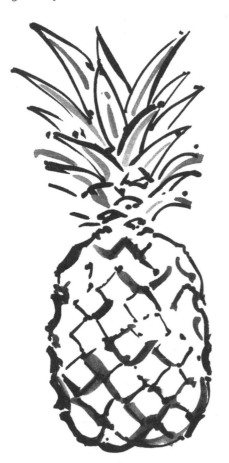

86 WAIT IT OUT

Often when people do a detox – particularly a three-day version, which is common with busy lifestyles – the skin can get worse before it gets better. Don't give up, though – your skin is the last organ to respond, so wait it out if you can.

87 PICK YOUR VARIETY

Fresh fruit is a major part of any detox diet, whether juicing, smoothies or the fruit itself. But some varieties contain far more fruit than others – look for old world varieties of apple, orange, pear and plum, which are not cultivated to be sweeter. Wherever you can, opt for sour-tasting fruit.

88 SMOKERS' DETOX TEA

Take a tablespoon of eucalyptus leaves and steep in a glass of boiling water; strain and add a tablespoon of glycerin and a tablespoon of honey. Drink around 50 ml (2fl oz) of the mixture four times a day for a week when you first quit smoking to help reduce cravings and detoxify naturally.

89 FLUSH YOUR LIVER

Squeeze the juice of a grapefruit and a lemon into a glass and dilute with filtered water. Add the juice of one clove of garlic, a knob of fresh ginger and a touch of extra virgin olive oil. Stir and sip slowly for a liver cleansing detox drink.

90 WAIVE THE WHEAT

A good starting point for detoxing is to cut out wheat, including bread, biscuits, cakes and pasta. Instead opt for bread and foods made from oats, rice, rye and spelt flour, or do away with bread products completely if you can.

91 DETOX WITH OATS

Take a tablespoon of ground oats (ground oats work better than oatmeal, but oatmeal may be substituted) and soak overnight in boiled water. The next morning, boil, allow to cool, divide into three and store in an airtight container. Consume one of these mini-drinks two hours after your three daily meals to help rid the body of toxins.

92 DO AWAY WITH DAIRY

Most detoxes advocate cutting out most of your dairy intake, including milk, cheese, ice cream and cream. Small amounts of butter and eggs are fine, but try replacing milk with soy, rice or oat milk products instead.

93 AVOID BACON AND HAM

Instead of choosing bacon and ham and other cured, smoked or dried meats, which contain lots of salt and sulphites, go for fresher meats such as chicken and beef, which are unpreserved. That way, you can be sure you're getting the maximum effects.

94 DRINK UP

Make up a liver-cleansing morning drink to replace your cappuccino. Mix the juice of half a fresh lemon, a pinch of cayenne pepper and a drizzle of honey or maple syrup. Top up with hot water for an energy-giving boost to the start of your day.

95 GET ALLIUM CLEAN

Allium vegetables – such as onions, garlic, shallots, leeks and chives – are great detox choices because their high levels of allicin boost production of glutathione, the body's natural detoxifier. For best results, consume raw or slightly cooked.

96 CHEW THE CUD

Grasses are a good choice for detoxification because they contain high levels of chlorophyll, which boost your blood cells' ability to carry oxygen and can therefore increase oxygenation and reduce inflammation.

get your beauty sleep

97 SLEEP YOURSELF HEALTHY

It's no coincidence that the expression "beauty sleep" exists. Sleep is the body's time to replenish and renew itself, and if you don't get enough sleep then your skin will suffer first, becoming dry, sensitive and prone to breakouts. Having to drag yourself out of bed in the morning and falling asleep within five minutes of going to bed at night are both signs you're not getting enough shut-eye.

98 SLEEP EASY

Did you know that for each hour of sleep you lose each night, your stress levels could increase by over 10 per cent? Stress increases glucocorticoids, which can increase skin problems such as acne, so it's important to get enough sleep. Keeping your bedroom cool at night is a great way to help you drop off.

99 TOASTY TOOTSIES

One of the best ways to help your body cool down as you go to bed at night is to wear a pair of loose-fitting bed socks. Having warm feet tricks your body's thermostat into slightly lowering its temperature, which gives a better night's sleep. For a luxurious feel, apply foot cream under your socks.

100 KEEP IT REGULAR

Many people who have trouble sleeping have erratic time schedules. Aim to go to bed and get up at roughly the same time every day, which will help train your body's rhythms into a daily schedule and make you more likely to sleep when your head hits the pillow.

101 SSHHHHHHH!

One of the worst culprits for sleep deprivation is a noisy bedroom. If you live near a road, street or railway make sure your windows are double-glazed or well insulated to help reduce noise, or invest in some ear plugs to help shut out any distractions.

102 BE A LAVENDER GIRL

Sprinkling a few drops of lavender oil on your pillow, or on a handkerchief near your bed, can help you sleep as the herb is linked to restfulness and helps your body feel calm and sleepy.

103 DIM THE LIGHTS

We naturally fall into a light sleep several times during the night. To help you sleep smoothly through this, make your room as dark as possible so the light won't encourage you to wake up. If it's impossible to darken your room (black-out blinds are useful for this), then wear a silk eye mask instead.

104 SOME LIKE IT HOT

Although it's best to steer clear of coffee and tea before bed, herbal teas like camomile and peppermint can relax your system and help you settle down more easily. Milky drinks (except hot chocolate) also encourage sleep because they line your stomach and contain a variety of slow-release sugars. Drink them warm for greatest effect.

105 KEEP IT MODERATE

Research shows that people who exercise regularly and those who spend some time outside every day have fewer sleep problems, but be careful of exercising late at night. If you must exert yourself close to bedtime, choose moderate exercise such as yoga or swimming.

106 FIND A PASSION

Passion flower is thought to help promote good sleep habits – drink an infusion of the petals, or use the dried flowers to help scent your bedroom. Other good herbs to try are valerian (seek medical advice before using this if you're on other medication), lemon verbena and lime flower.

107 REDUCE YOUR SUGAR INTAKE

Eating food and drink that's high in sugar (including alcohol and caffeine) in the evening can cause you to wake during the night as your body's systems deal with the subsequent sugar low. Aim for low GI foods for your evening meal and avoid sugar, caffeine and "treat" snacks after 6 pm.

108 BATH BEFORE BED

A warm bath will gently warm and relax you. In addition, the reduction in body temperature about 15 minutes after your bath is a great way to mimic the body's natural sleep rhythms and encourage slumber. It's good for skin too, as cleansing and applying cream means your skin has the whole night to soak up the benefits.

109 THINK YOURSELF CALM

Spend a few minutes every night before you turn out the light doing some deep breathing while concentrating on reducing any areas of tension in your body. Listen to music as you do so to help shut out other thoughts and use mental images of a favourite place or moment (an idyllic holiday spot, for example) as a way of helping you regain feelings of relaxation and wellbeing before you drift off.

110 TRY TRYPTOPHAN

Foods containing the amino acid tryptophan are thought to encourage sleep by boosting the brain's natural sleepy chemicals. Turkey, bananas and wholemeal bread are all good tryptophan trips, and may combine with vitamin B (found in bananas, avocados and astragalus) to help reduce adrenal stress.

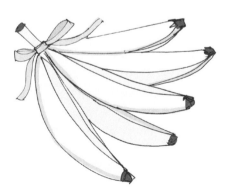

give up smoking

111 LEAVE LONGER BETWEEN BLASTS

As well as introducing toxins to the body, which it has to divert vitamins away from the skin to deal with, cigarettes also contain nicotine, which reduces blood flow to the dermis (where new skin cells are generated), leaving skin looking sallow and lifeless. If you must smoke, leave as long as possible between exposures – for instance, only smoke for one or two hours a day.

112 THE FUTURE'S ORANGE

Oranges are a great choice for getting rid of niggly cravings as they contain natural compounds which help rid the body of nicotine compounds, reducing physical cravings, and their citrus smell and taste delivers an energy punch. The acidity also helps with mental cravings, by "filling" the tastebuds. If you don't like oranges, try grapes, dried pineapple or mango instead.

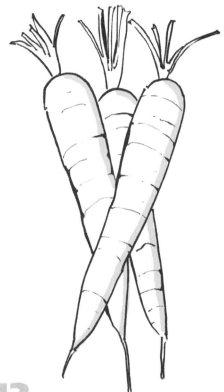

113 BE A JUICE BABY

Vegetable juices are a great way to fight off cigarette cravings and they contain high levels of vitamin C, which is thought to help reduce nicotine in the system and boost skin health. Carrot, celery and pumpkin juice are all good choices. Combine with a sweeter fruit juice such as orange or pineapple if you find the taste unpalatable.

114 BE A HONEY

One of the best ways to beat off cigarette cravings is to have a spoonful of honey. The taste is strong enough to mask cravings and the complex sugars give your blood sugar levels a slow lift, reducing the severity of cravings by stimulating your brain's "feel-good" receptors.

115 TASTE SOME LIQ-OUR

Chewing liquorice is a good way of fighting off cigarette cravings as the herb is both sweet and soothing – it contains natural relaxation properties that help induce calmness in the middle of a craving. It fills your mouth with a satisfying "full" taste, leaving you less likely to cave in.

116 SALT YOUR TONGUE

For the first three days after you give up smoking you can help fight off cravings for a cigarette by using salt – simply dip a finger in salt and apply to the very tip of the tongue when you feel a craving coming on. Follow after a few minutes, when the craving has passed, with a glass of water.

117 GET SMOOTH

US studies have found that smokers in their forties have as many wrinkles on their face as non-smokers in their sixties because smoking breaks down the main structural protein in the skin, collagen. Smokers are also far more likely to have psoriasis, especially women. The best thing you can do for your skin is to give up completely.

118 LIKE LYCOPENE

If you are an ex-smoker, eat lots of tomatoes (preferably cooked), which contain high levels of lycopene to help repair the damage you have done to your skin by smoking, or take a lycopene supplement if you don't like them. Exfoliate twice a week to stimulate collagen production and drink enough water to keep skin hydrated.

119 SAVE YOUR PENNIES

Put away all the money you would have spent on cigarettes when you cut down or quit and buy yourself something healthy, like a facial or body treatment, to make the most of your newly healthy skin.

hydration tips

120 GET SOME SPARKLE

It's the sugar, sweeteners, flavourings and colours in fizzy drinks that make them so bad for your skin, and general health, not the fact that they're fizzy. In fact, some studies have shown that carbonated mineral water can be better than tap water for reaping health benefits. It's especially good at parties or evenings out if you're trying to avoid alcohol.

121 SET YOUR ALARM

Many people who lead busy lives forget to drink enough water then gulp down two or three glasses at once when they finally remember. If this sounds like you, why not set your phone or computer alarm to remind you every hour and a half to two hours, then drink a small glass of water at each alarm.

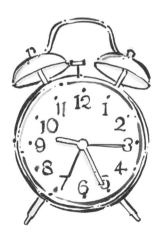

122 GET STEAMY

If you suffer from dry skin, especially in the winter, try investing in a humidifier for your bedroom, or for other rooms in your home if you spend lots of time in them. The extra moisture it creates in the air can help your skin avoid losing too much moisture and also reduces dryness.

123 GO FRESH

Wherever possible, choose fresh fruit rather than dried. This will not only help rehydrate your body by adding precious water (in an unpolluted form), but also help regulate your sugar levels, as people who eat dried fruit tend to consume more sugar before they feel full.

124 GO HERBAL

It's not just fruit that can flavour water – a sugar-free way to give your water a bit of added oomph is to crush up some herbs, such as rosemary, mint, basil or thyme. Sprinkle them into the water, then strain before drinking. Or make up some herbal ice cubes instead.

125 MAKE IT A HALF

Get into the habit of drinking half a glass of water before every meal or snack during the day – you'll have taken in nearly half of your daily allowance without even thinking about it. Also food is usually better-absorbed if mixed with water so you're getting double the benefits.

126 BE A COCO-NUT

Coconut water (taken from green coconuts) is a great choice as it nourishes and rehydrates without sugar. It's virtually fat-free but stacked full of potassium, amino acids and electrolytes which allow the body to rehydrate quickly and efficiently.

127 GET MUSICAL

If you're exercising to music, use your playlist to remind you to keep hydrated by taking a small drink at the end of every song – that way you will make sure you keep your fluid levels topped up and don't risk dehydration.

128 DO YOUR CALCULATIONS

If you want to know how much water you lose from your body during normal activity, do a weight test – weigh yourself at 8 am and then again at 10 am. Make sure you don't eat or drink anything during this time and the weight you have lost will be pure water. A loss of 500 g (1 lb) is equivalent to 600 ml (1 pint) of water.

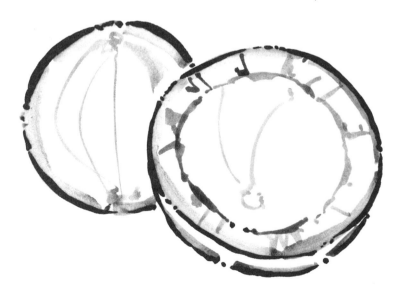

129 SEE YOUR PEE

Your urine is a great signpost to how dehydrated your body is. Light and straw-coloured is perfect – if it's totally clear, you're drinking too much and if it's dark, like tea or beer, you need to drink more. Aim for 1.5–2 litres (2½–3½ pints) a day if you have an active lifestyle.

130 SAVOUR THE FLAVOUR

Some people simply don't like the taste of water. If that's you, try flavouring it with a couple of slices of fruit such as lemon, orange, peach or lime and adding some ice. Or simply dilute pure fruit juice. It's a much better choice than cordial, which often contains high levels of sugar.

131 PINCH AN INCH

A good indicator as to whether your skin is dehydrated is the skin on the back of your hands, which is fairly thin and therefore prone to losing moisture. Pinch the skin, hold for three seconds, and then release – if skin is hydrated, it will bounce back into shape.

132 USE A FILTER

Even if you're fastidiously drinking six to eight glasses of water a day, if you're relying on poor-quality water you could be missing out on health benefits. To get the best hydration, filter your tap water or choose mineral water. If you spend a lot of time at home, consider fitting a whole house water filter or under-sink filter to make sure all your water is clear.

133 ICE IT UP

Why not make up some fruit ice cubes – freeze a mixture of half juice, half water in an ice-cube tray. Pop one in the top of your glass of water – it's a great way to flavour your drink while minimizing sugar intake.

134 BE PREPARED

You're much more likely to remember to drink the right amount of water if it's visible – try taking a small jug to work and keep it on your desk to refill your glass. Aim to drink one jug before lunch and another afterwards by sipping throughout the day.

135 JOIN A BAND

A great way to make sure you're drinking enough is to use the "rubber band" technique. If you plan to have six glasses of water a day, for instance, put six rubber bands around the bottom of the glass or your wrist in the morning and remove one every time you refill your glass, aiming to remove all the bands during the day. Or you could use bangles and move them from one wrist to the other.

136 GO HOT

In the winter, a hot drink such as tea or coffee is far more appealing than cold water. Mix one-quarter cold water with three-quarters water from the kettle (to ensure it's not too hot) and sip away. Try to alternate hot water with caffeinated drinks.

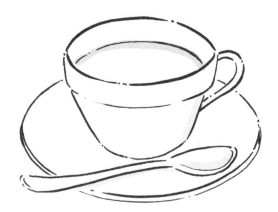

beat stress & anxiety

137 ADD A DROP

Smell is the most emotionally linked of our senses so if you like the fragrance of a product, chances are you'll believe it will do you more good. If you have a favourite smell which really helps you relax, like rose or lavender, add a drop or two to unscented products to provide the benefits of the smell, as well as your product. Doing this at night will help you relax before bed, or try first thing in the morning to carry you through the day.

138 BREATHE AWAY STRESS

Deep breathing is not only good for helping to reduce stress levels, it also helps reduce stress and anxiety by reducing levels of stress hormone. Find a comfortable position, close your eyes and breathe in for one, two, three and out for one, two, three, four, five. Repeat three to 10 times.

139 CALM DOWN, DEAR

Stress can make inflammatory conditions such as psoriasis, rosacea and acne worse and cause other skin problems, like breakouts, dullness, blushing and flushing, hives and perspiration. The more it accumulates, the worse things get. If you feel stressed, take action sooner rather than later (see below) to keep your skin smooth and healthy.

140 GET NEEDLED

Acupuncture is a great way to help reduce anxiety and stress, and it's been shown to have direct effects in reducing the symptoms of eczema, too. If you don't like needles, try acupressure massage instead.

141 HAVE A TREATMENT

Cosmetic solutions to bad skin, such as AHA rejuvenation treatments, do much to improve outward appearance but they can also affect wellbeing from the inside. Feeling better inside reduces neuropeptides being released from the nerve endings, which can help skin appear smoother and healthier.

142 GET YOGIC

Taking up a gentle, stress-relieving activity like walking, swimming or yoga can help reduce stress levels and gives your skin a chance to get back its healthy glow; it also reduces inflammation and sensitivity. Aim for three times a week for best results.

143 PAMPER YOURSELF

It's official: spending your well-earned cash on beauty treatments has benefits that reach far beyond the treatment itself. The feeling of wellbeing can last several days or even weeks, regulating hormones and giving the skin a chance to shine. If you can't afford salon treatments, why not organize a home spa night with a friend and take turns to pamper each other?

144 KEEP A JOURNAL

If you have too many thoughts running around in your head, which stop you relaxing and unwinding, keeping a journal could help. Get into the habit of spending five to 10 minutes a day writing down how you feel. It's been shown to reduce stress and anxiety.

healthy skin, night & day

145 DAY AND NIGHT

Always use separate day and night creams. The day creams are designed to quickly absorb into the skin and not interfere with make-up application whereas night creams are more emollient and intended for bare skin. Products especially designed for overnight use are packed with vitamins and usually have a specific delivery system that enables the skin to maximize the extra regeneration of cells that occurs during night-time.

146 GO BACK TO SLEEP

Try not to sleep on your stomach as this can contribute to wrinkles as the pillow pushes against your face, neck and décolleté. Sleeping curled up on your side in the foetal position creates wrinkles and creases on the side of your face where the skin is at its thinnest. Lying on your back is a good choice as gravity pushes skin backwards, like a mini-overnight facelift.

147 ASSESS TO CLEANSE BEST

Your first step in the morning should be to take a good look in the mirror. Note any dry patches on cheeks or oiliness in the T-zone. Hormones, seasons, environment and diet can all impact on your skin and will be evident – you can then adjust your regime accordingly.

148 FALL IN GLOVE

Overnight is a great time to give your hands a bit of TLC, especially if you lead an active life. Apply hand cream before you go to sleep and if skin feels extremely dry, invest in a pair of light cotton gloves to maximize the moisturizing effects.

149 PILLOW PRESSURE

Burying your face in a pillow puts pressure on your skin, which in turn reduces circulation. Over time the wear and tear this causes will break down collagen and cause lines and wrinkles. Switch to silk, satin or a high thread count cotton to minimize friction on facial skin.

150 KEEP IT LIGHT

Every skin type needs a daily moisturizer,
so know the one suitable for you.
Lightweight gels and simple moisturizers
are good for young and sensitive skins.

151 SLEEP AWAY WRINKLES

Keep neck stretched upwards by sleeping
on a high-density contour foam pillow
that conforms to your shape and provides
maximum support to help prevent sleep
wrinkles forming on face and neck.

152 FIRM AND MOISTURIZE

For very dry or mature skin, a firming
serum or treatment applied underneath
a moisturizer gives an added boost to
daytime skin, replicating the youthful
shine of younger skin beautifully.

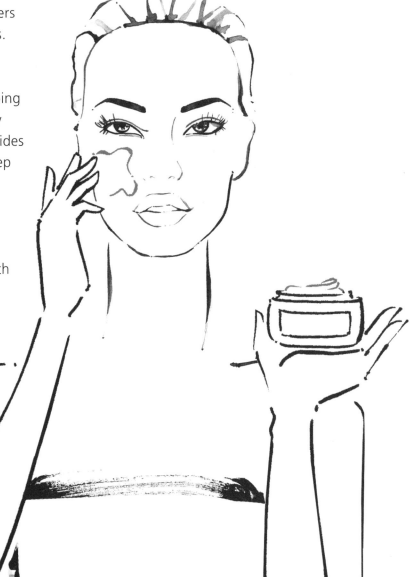

choosing products for your skin type

153 BE A HONEY

A honey face mask is a good choice for oily skin, adding moisture without increasing oiliness. The anti-bacterial properties of honey also reduce inflammation and risk of infection. Mash up a tablespoon of honey (use the famously antiseptic manuka honey if skin is prone to spots) and a banana with a teaspoon of lemon juice. Apply to the face, leave for five to 15 minutes and rinse with warm water.

154 HIT THE SPOT

Just because you get a few spots, that doesn't mean you have acne. Acne is characterized by inflammation of the glands under the skin of an area of the face, rather than isolated spots. The skin looks red and sore, with clogged and blocked pores, and it's usually related to hormones. People with genuine acne should seek medical help.

155 DITCH THE DETERGENTS

If you have dry skin, choose products that don't contain detergents and don't use soap to cleanse your skin. Instead, choose cream or balm cleansers and use a special night cream to add extra moisture.

156 HANDS OFF OILY SKIN

Touching, stroking and facial massage stimulates the skin's oil glands to produce more sebum, which is the last thing oily skin needs. So, if you want to dry out oily areas, keep your hands away from your face.

157 TIGHTEN UP

If your skin is oily, products designed to tighten pores can be useful to help improve its general appearance and reduce shine. Choose masks containing clay to draw out impurities and use a toner regularly.

158 STAY SHADY

If you have dry skin, the sun is more of an enemy for you than other skin types as it causes dryness and flaking. Wind is another culprit, so your dry skin will thank you if you avoid extremes of weather and seek shade from the wind and sun wherever you can.

159 GO MINERAL

Mineral make-up is a great choice for skin which is prone to clogging and breakouts as it encourages impurities to leave the skin and allows you to wear make-up without the risk of clogging or blocking up pores. Be sure to remove it at night, though, to give skin a total breather.

160 DRYNESS ON TAP

If your skin is really dry, and feels tight after washing, avoid tap water for a while – the chemicals it often contains can be harsh on already-dry skin. Try mineral water instead, or use an alcohol-free cleansing lotion or cream.

161 GET SOME TONE

Just because you have dry skin, this doesn't mean you have to ditch the toner but make sure you use a really gentle version that doesn't contain alcohol or other astringents.

162 THAT'S THE RUB

If the skin on your face and body is dry, avoid rubbing with a towel after a bath or shower. Instead pat gently to leave a layer of moisture on the skin while you apply your cream or butter to help boost humidity.

163 OIL THE CREAKS

If dry skin feels tight and creaky after you cleanse or wash it, swap your moisturizing cream for an oil-based lotion or oil, which can help boost the skin's moisture levels by replacing lost moisture straight away.

salon secrets

164 ASK AHEAD

If you're visiting a salon for a treatment you haven't had before, don't rely on them to tell you everything you need to know. Do your research about what to expect in advance and be sure to ask your therapist any questions before treatment begins.

165 BE SENSITIVE

If you have sensitive skin and you know some of your triggers, make sure you tell your therapist so they can choose the right products. If you're at all worried, pop into the salon the day before and ask to be given a patch test.

166 UNPLUG YOURSELF

If you're having a treatment that involves an electric current, like Muscle Toning, make sure you remove piercings all over your body, even if they're not in the same area. If your piercings are hidden (i.e. tummy button or genitals), be sure to tell your therapist so they don't interfere with treatment.

167 DRESS FOR SUCCESS

Whatever treatment you're having, some clothes will help and others will hinder your therapist from doing their best. If you're not sure, check before you go, but generally speaking, cotton briefs, boxers or Y-fronts are best, and loose, comfortable clothing.

168 CHECK THE SHELVES

In the absence of a register or grading system for salons, use clues to work out whether or not a salon is reputable. If they use a well-known brand such as Eve Lom, Aromatherapy Associates, Elemis or Clarins, they are likely to have had to reach minimum requirements. Check also for a certificate of insurance and that the salon has a public liability component.

169 TELL ON THE TINGLE

If, during any sort of face or body treatment, your skin starts to tingle, itch or feel strange in any way, or if you feel something doesn't seem quite right, mention it to your therapist straight away so they can ensure you're getting the best care.

170 IMAGE-INE

If you're visiting a salon for semi-permanent tattoos (like eye make-up, lip liner or eyebrow colouring), make sure you check your therapist's work before you agree to anything. Ask to see images and check they're actually that therapist's work and not just generic brand images.

171 ALLERGY ALERT

If you're allergic to shellfish, make sure you tell your beauty therapist because many face products contain ground shells as an added ingredient, which could cause an allergic reaction, redness or swelling.

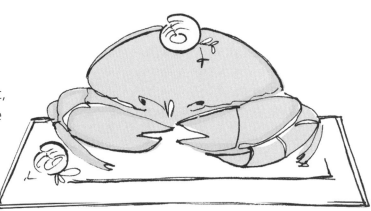

172 BE HONEST

Your salon should ask you several screening questions before any treatment, but do offer up any information that might be useful to them, even if it's not on the questionnaire. If you're pregnant, breastfeeding, menopausal, on medication or have any physical ailments, it can help your therapist to make sure you get the right treatment and they don't do anything dangerous.

173 SETTLE DOWN

Don't worry about going to sleep during your treatment – most therapists consider this a compliment. But it's a shame to sleep through the whole treatment and miss out on the enjoyment of it, so try to get a good night's sleep before your appointment or take a short power nap beforehand instead.

174 SPEAK UP

Before starting your treatment, your therapist should tell you exactly what's going to happen while you are there. If there's anything you don't like the sound of (like oil in your hair for a facial), speak up immediately.

professional treatments

175 MICRODERMABRASION

This skin-booster uses aluminium oxide particles to slough off the outermost layers to leave the complexion brighter and even out colour and tone. There are home-based alternatives, but professional is best to reduce redness and avoid irritation post-treatment.

176 BE PREPARED

Instead of being used after wrinkles appear, many experts now suggest Botox as a preventative measure to stop lines appearing in the first place. Treatment in your thirties or forties is increasingly popular.

177 SMOOTH SPOTS

A good salon choice for spotty or greasy skins, smoothbeam lasers target oil glands and slows down oil production. This in turn helps prevent spots and blackheads and stimulates collagen production, which can tighten pores.

178 LOOK YOUNGER WITH MESOTHERAPY

Mesotherapy, in which vitamins, minerals and antioxidants are injected into the middle layer of the skin, is said to improve skin quality and vitality by replenishing it with essential vitamins that occur naturally within the cells. The vitamins A, E, C, D and B create firmness, clarity and smoothness in the skin.

179 WAITING GAME

Botox can take four to 10 days for the treatment to take full effect, which means it's hard to see exactly what the end result will be. To avoid the frozen look, ask for minimal amounts of the treatment.

180 KNOW YOUR AURA

We once had to visit salons for light and laser treatments, but now companies like Philips are launching at-home laser treatments complete with consultations when you buy the product to ensure you use it correctly. Based on Fraxel technology, a skin resurfacing laser treatment designed to target depths up to 1.6 mm, the RéAura device beams microscopic laser beams to resurface skin.

181 GO SUPERSONIC

Some products are now introducing sonic technology into the home for advanced cleansing. Clarisonic products offer up to six times better make-up removal than manual and they also come with different attachments for normal, sensitive, deep pore and delicate cleansing.

182 KNOW YOUR PRODUCTS

If you suffer from acne, some of the hydrating and oil-based lotions in a typical facial could cause your skin to break out. Look for words like "clarifying" or "purifying", which are designed for acne-prone or oily skin.

183 REQUEST SAMPLES

After a facial, ask your therapist if they can give you any trial samples to take home with you. Each product sample should last a couple of days, enabling you to extend the benefits and you can also decide whether to invest in the products long term.

184 AVOID EXTRACTION

Extractors are made of inflexible metal so it's hard to judge the right amount of pressure to perform an extraction without scarring. Ask your facialist to use her gauze- or cotton-wrapped fingertips instead.

185 GET BLASTED

If your skin needs serious resurfacing attention for deep lines, consult an expert about using a fractional CO_2 laser – it has deep effects, but requires two to three weeks of total "down time" afterwards as the skin heals.

186 AVOID THE STEAM

If you have eczema or rosacea, ask your facialist to skip the steam step of the facial (which for normal skin helps soften and open pores). To avoid exacerbating the condition, use a warm cloth instead.

facial peels

187 PREPARE FOR PRODUCTS

Facial peels with glycolic, salicylic or lactic acids are not just for ageing skin – everyone's skin can look firmer and smoother, and a mild peel is a great way to strip back skin, ready to benefit most from other skincare products. Ask your therapist for advice.

188 CHECK THE SMALL PRINT

One of the most important things about home facial peels is that you must always remember to read the label. Don't assume that the instructions will be the same for different types and brands, and make sure you follow the advice carefully.

189 LESS IS MORE

The glow that peels give your skin can be addictive, but remember they actually take away the top layers of skin, and that's the layer for sun cream to adhere to and to protect against pollution and other irritants. Avoid having a salon peel more than once a month or an at-home peel more than once a week.

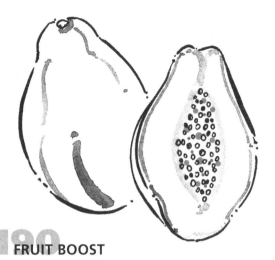

180 FRUIT BOOST

Often facial peels now have added fruit and vegetables to deliver an antioxidant boost as well as the traditional "peel" action, which dissolves the glue holding cells together to slough off the topmost layers. Superfood additives such as pumpkin, blueberries and papaya are common ingredients.

181 TAKE CARE IN THE SUN

Because peels are designed to resurface the skin, they leave the surface layers less protected against sun damage, so it's doubly important that you follow aftercare instructions carefully, including using a sunscreen every day.

182 GO MEDICAL

Certain facial peels (particularly those for acne scarring and pigmentation) are only available on prescription, but they can have amazing results. Consult a dermatologist about medical peel products; Obagi is a recommended brand available globally on prescription.

183 SET YOUR EXPECTATIONS

Peels can work really well to help smooth and exfoliate skin, but they only work on the top layers of skin, so don't expect the same deep-reaching results as laser resurfacing. Also, home peels have lower concentrations than salon treatments, so it's worth visiting a salon every so often to get a stronger effect.

184 KNOW YOUR LEVEL

There are different levels of chemical peels, with vastly different results – if you want exfoliation, choose a superficial or light chemical peel; for pigment irregularities such as melasma and age spots, it's medium strength. Deep strength is used to remove wrinkles in the deep layers of skin. Generally, if you want more than a superficial peel, you need to visit a medical provider.

195 GLOVE UP

When performing a facial peel at home, it's a good idea to wear gloves to prevent the "peel" from affecting your hands as well as your face. If you plan to use peels regularly, invest in a box of disposable latex gloves so you can wear a clean pair every time.

196 GET SOME VASELINE

Because they are usually liquid, chemical peels can often spread over the skin to areas you are not planning on treating – steal a trick from the pros and delineate the boundary with Vaseline first to prevent it from spreading.

197 PEEL OFF THE LAYERS

Technological advances mean you can now get similar results at home to those achieved with a medically administered chemical peel. Over-the-counter "peel" kits contain chemicals such as glycolic acid that lift off the top layers of skin to reveal a brighter complexion. They usually have a two- or three-part process: the acid solution, an agent to calm skin and stop the action, followed by a moisturizer.

198 KEEP IT STERILE

When you're using food items for facial skincare, be sure to use clean apparatus and sterile pots (washing in a dishwasher and leaving to dry is good enough). Before any treatment, wash hands really well and consider a patch test if you're using a new ingredient: apply a bit to the inside of your wrist, wait 20 minutes and if there's no reaction you should be fine. If you feel any discomfort, remove immediately.

at-home treatments

199 GIVE SKIN A FEAST

Skin is the last organ to reap the benefits of all the good things you eat, so often there's precious little nourishment left, even with a relatively good diet. Choose face treatments high in essential minerals such as calcium, magnesium and zinc to give it a boost.

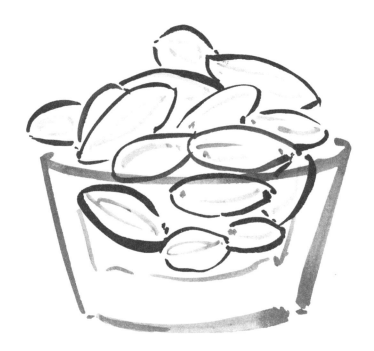

200 SKIN CLEARER

Almonds are a gentle cleanser and they're great for removing impurities too. Grind up a tablespoon of almonds (or use ready-ground) and mix together with a tablespoon each of egg white and lemon or lime juice (use lemon if your skin is prone to oil; lime if prone to dryness or combination). Apply to face for five to 10 minutes then rinse thoroughly.

201 TAKE CARE

Are you allergic to nuts? Make sure you avoid oils and products containing them as well. If you're at all unsure whether you might have a problem, do a patch test on your wrist or inner arm first to be sure.

202 SCRUB UP WELL

Everyone waxes lyrical about the benefits of exfoliating, but there is a danger in overdoing it – taking away too much leaves skin unprotected and can cause dryness, itching and irritation in the upper layers. For best results, keep it to once or twice a week.

203 GET CITRUS CLEAR

Being a natural exfoliant, lemon is great for getting rid of blackheads. Mix equal amounts of lemon juice and rosewater together and apply to the affected area. Leave for 10 minutes, then rinse or cleanse off. If you're short on time, simply cut a lemon in half and rub the flesh over the skin you want to treat, wait a few minutes and rinse.

204 PEACHY CHEEKS

There's no need to mix up a home-made face cream for a fruit boost – simply cut a peach in half, remove the stone and rub the inside onto your cheeks to boost vitamin and mineral levels and hydration. Leave for 10 minutes to half an hour and rinse off with warm water.

205 SPOT IT

Fruits contain natural acids, which can help reduce the appearance of blemishes and boost skin regeneration. Use a clean finger to dab a few drops of apple, orange, melon or cucumber juice onto blemishes to encourage them to heal naturally.

206 GET YOUR OATS

Oats are not only good for breakfast – they have great soothing abilities for dry, sensitive or problem skin, especially on the face. Add ground oats to home-made creams and masks, or combine with natural yogurt or fruit juice for a quick skin booster. Simply apply to skin, leave five to 20 minutes and then wash off.

207 GO FACIAL

Cucumber isn't just good for refreshing tired eyes – grate, juice or blend up a cucumber and use as a face mask to help hydrate skin and prevent pimples, dryness and wrinkles. Apply with clean fingertips and wipe or rinse off with lukewarm water after 15 minutes.

208 ADD YOGURT

Yogurt is a great natural moisturizer for the skin and, because of its helpful bacteria, it also helps to reduce blemishes. For the best effects, choose live natural yogurt. Add to home-made face creams and masks for immediate use, or use on its own for a 30-minute skin booster. Make sure that you rinse well afterwards.

209 EGG-CELLENT RESULTS

Egg white is a wonderful facial product as it contains naturally high levels of albumin protein, which helps the skin store water and prevents dehydration. Mix an egg white with a spoonful of live natural yogurt (which contains lactic acid to tighten and brighten skin) for a quick facial booster.

210 CLEANSE WITH LIME

With high levels of vitamins and antioxidants, lime juice is a natural cleanser; it can also be less harsh than lemon. Squeeze the juice of a lime into a cup of warm water and use to cleanse your face with a face cloth.

211 GET CORNY

Mix up some cornmeal or oatmeal with water until you get a thick, but smooth paste. Use as a scrub to exfoliate the skin on your face, neck and décolletage. Massage in long, gentle strokes rather than scrubbing, then rinse.

212 GET SOLUBLE

Aspirin contains a form of salicylic acid, which is the active ingredient in many acne treatments, making it a good choice for problem skin treatments at home. Dissolve three or four soluble aspirin tablets in warm water to make a thick paste and add either a few drops of tea tree oil (if you have problem skin) or aloe vera gel (if your skin needs some TLC). Apply to the face using gentle circular movements and rinse off after a few minutes.

213 GET MILKY

Milk of magnesia might seem an unlikely choice for facial skincare, but it's an excellent way to calm and soothe problem skin and breakouts because it contains high levels of magnesium hydroxide, which absorbs oil and has antibacterial properties. Apply a small amount to skin on a cotton ball or pad, leave to dry and rinse off.

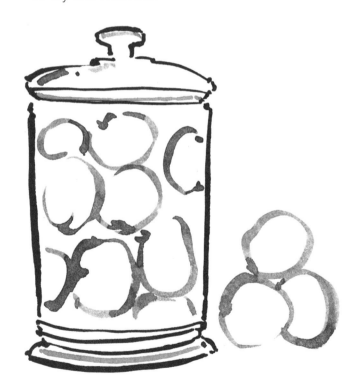

good habits

214 FACIALIZE

Make every night a beautiful one by incorporating a mini-facial into your bedtime routine. Simply adding a few extra strokes along your cheeks and up toward eyes can help stimulate blood flow, or splash face with cold water before applying night cream.

215 TOUCH OF CLOTH

Using a muslin or towelling facecloth to wash your face morning and night helps keep dead skin sloughed off and your skin feeling fresh and clean as it gently exfoliates as you wash. Make sure you don't scrub your face, though as this could lead to thread veins or red patches.

216 FINISH WELL

If you didn't exfoliate before a mask, finish by removing the mask using a warm, wet facecloth in gentle circular movements. This acts as a gentle exfoliant to leave skin instantly brighter and clearer-looking. Do not use a scrub or product exfoliator at this stage.

217 STEAM AWAY IMPURITIES

For a quick, deep cleanse, pour boiling water into a bowl. Sprinkle with lemon juice and rose petals, then cover your head with a towel and hold your face over the bowl. The steam will invigorate you, aid in respiration and helps loosen blackheads. Cleanse afterwards and follow with a cool-water rinse to close pores.

218 CHECK BEHIND YOUR EARS

Always remember to use anti-ageing serums and moisturizers behind your ears and the back of your neck to keep hidden areas well hydrated and help prevent skin from sagging.

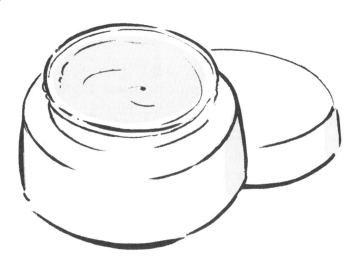

219 SLEEP CLEAN

It's an old adage, but never go to bed with your make-up on. It prevents the skin from shedding and breathing, and may even cause blemishes and/or blackheads to appear.

220 NOW WASH YOUR HANDS

Always make sure your hands are clean before you touch your face. When applying foundation, use a sponge or brush to give a velvety look and avoid oil production.

221 CLEANSE BEFORE YOU COVER

You wouldn't polish a dirty floor and neither should you apply a mask to a dirty face. You'll only get the full benefits if you apply the mask to cleansed skin, which allows your face to absorb more of the ingredients in the mask.

222 BEWARE OF OVERCLEANSING

Overcleansing is a major cause of sensitive skin as it strips the underlayers of its natural protective properties. Be sure to use a cleanser that's right for your skin type and don't overdo it.

223 TIP OF THE DAY

When cleansing, many people forget the tip of their nose, which can then become oily or greasy. Use small circular movements to make sure you get your whole nose clean!

224 CLEANSE BEFORE YOU COLOUR

Before applying your make-up in the morning, make sure you thoroughly cleanse your face and apply moisturizer to even out the skin first.

225 POST-MASK MOISTURE BOOST

Always moisturize directly after using a mask, unless the mask is a leave-on product and you are instructed to rub in the residue. With dead skin cells sloughed off and pores unclogged, your moisturizer will sink in more deeply and have more penetrative results.

226 KEEP YOUR HAIR OFF

Keep hair clean and away from your face to avoid making skin greasy, especially overnight when it can rub against skin as you sleep and cause spots and blemishes.

237 DON'T BE A WASHOUT

If you have oily skin, the worst thing you can do is to overwash it or use a harsh cleanser, as these actually encourage more production of oils in the skin and might make you spottier. Avoid alcohol-based products that strip the skin and opt for lotions rather than heavy creams.

228 GET OFF YOUR SOAP BOX!

Whatever your skin type, avoid using even mild bath soap on the sensitive skin of your face, neck and behind the ears, as this can leave skin feeling tight and drained. It may also cause redness and rashes. Choose a cleanser specially formulated for your face.

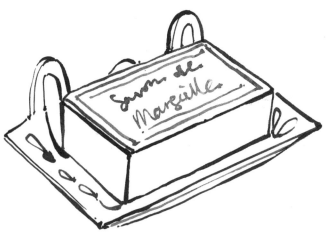

face masks

229 DO A PATCH TEST

Take care when using masks, especially if you have sensitive skin. Test a small amount of the mask on the area behind your ear and leave for 24 hours to see if there's a reaction. Always remove masks immediately if you feel any tingling or burning.

230 LAY IT ON THICK

Most home-made masks work best when coverage is generous, so don't be afraid to use a thicker application. This is one area when trying to skimp proves a false economy because the mask won't do as much for the skin if it's thin and you'll only be tempted to use it more often.

231 BE A SMOOTH-SKINNED HONEY

Honey and almond flour, mixed together into a paste, produces an excellent scrub for oily skin – honey has antiseptic properties and, like the almond flour, contains high levels of vitamins. The scrub's graininess makes it a gentle exfoliator.

232 WATERMELON CLEANSER

Make yourself a cleansing and clarifying face mask using watermelon, which clears the skin of blemishes and leaves it feeling fresh and clear. Apply the pure juice to your face, leave for 15 minutes and then splash with cold water to remove it.

233 MUD, GLORIOUS MUD

Oily skin responds well to clay- or mud-based masks, but never use them on dry skin – they are too harsh. If you suffer from an oily T-zone but dry cheeks, apply the mud mask only in the T-zone area and use a gentle moisturizing mask for your cheeks.

234 BREW UP A STORM

For oily skin, a brewer's yeast mask can help tone without drying out. Mix a teaspoon of brewer's yeast with enough natural yogurt to make a loose, thin mixture. Pat this thoroughly into the oily areas and leave to dry on the skin. After 15 to 20 minutes rinse off with warm water, then cool and blot dry.

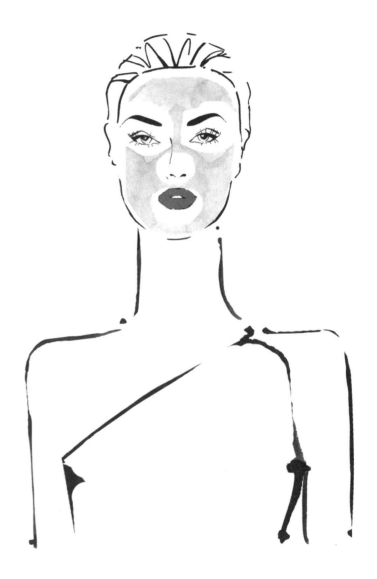

235 GO BANANAS

Banana is one of the best ingredients for an anti-wrinkle treatment because of the vitamins and minerals it contains and its smooth, soothing consistency. Mash two or three slices with a little milk, apply all over your face and leave for 15 to 20 minutes before rinsing off with warm water.

236 GRAPE BOOST

Forget expensive lotions – grape juice makes an excellent cleanser for any skin type. Simply split one or two large grapes, remove their pips and rub the flesh over your face and neck for an instant, antioxidant cleanser. Rinse off with cool water.

237 PACK IT WITH PETALS

Prepare a rose face mask by blending a handful of petals into a paste with a little milk and a tablespoon of honey, if desired. Apply to clean skin and leave for 15 to 25 minutes. Wash the paste off with plain water (no soap) and your complexion will be left smooth, soft and glowing.

238 PUT ON YOUR SANDALS

If your skin suffers from dryness, make a calming, rehydrating face cream with sandalwood paste (from healthfood shops), olive oil and honey. Add a touch of rose oil if your skin is extra-dry, or turmeric if you're prone to blackheads or breakouts.

239 USE BETA-CARROT-ENE

A beta-carotene carrot mask can work wonders for blemished complexions. Use a small, raw carrot blended to a smooth paste or boil in a little water and then mash it. Pat the mask all over the blemished areas and leave for 15 to 20 minutes. Rinse and pat dry.

240 GO NUTS

Some of the most beneficial oils for dry skin are avocados and almonds. Make up a nourishing mask by mashing a small avocado with a teaspoon of almond oil. Apply to the face and neck and leave for 10 to 20 minutes before rinsing off with warm water or a warm cloth. Give yourself an internal boost by snacking on any leftovers!

241 MIX UP A VITAMIN BLEND

Create a replenishing face mask with the flesh of one avocado, a little orange juice, honey, molasses and a few drops of camomile essential oil whizzed together in a blender to give your skin a vitamin boost.

242 TISSUES FOR DRY ISSUES

If your skin is extra-dry, masks for dry skin can be wiped away with a tissue so that a thin film of the moisture stays behind, quenching skin for hours afterwards. Be careful not to leave too much product, though, as it can clog pores.

243 GET YOUR OATS

Create a fabulously soothing and moisturizing oatmeal face mask by mixing together an egg yolk with a tablespoon of honey. Add enough smooth oatmeal to make a thick paste. Leave on for 10 minutes, or 15 minutes if your skin is very dry and needs a calming boost.

244 CUCUMBER REHYDRATOR

To gently rehydrate sensitive skin, combine half a cucumber (scooped out of its skin), one tablespoon of yogurt, a few strawberries and one teaspoon of honey. Apply to your face, allow to dry, then gently wipe off.

245 EGGS-ELEVEN

Eggs can be used to make masks to suit all skin types. Whipped and patted on the skin, an egg white tightens and tones. The whole egg, beaten, has softening properties as well. Add an egg to any mask for an "eggstra" treat!

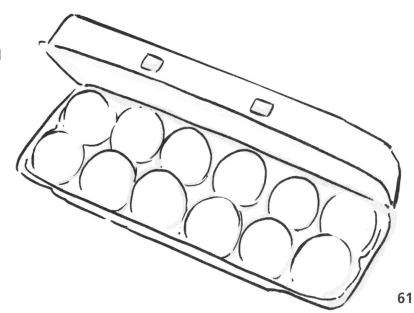

saunas & steaming

246 CLEAN UP

Before you do any sort of facial steaming at home, make sure your face is thoroughly cleansed. Boil the water in a kettle then leave for five to 10 minutes to cool so that it doesn't burn you. Tie or scrape back your hair and place a bowl somewhere you can sit comfortably for five to 10 minutes. Drape a towel over your head and slowly lower your face over the water until you feel the warmth of the steam (it should feel comfortable, not too hot). Finish off with cool or cold water and pay skin dry before applying a face mask or moisturizer.

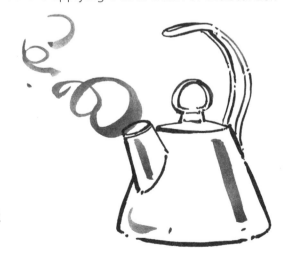

247 GET SOFT

If you have breakouts or acne, the heat of a sauna can help soften the acne cysts and thus help skin to heal and regenerate more quickly. Be careful if you suffer from thickened skin or clogged pores, though, as this could exacerbate swelling.

248 GO CAREFULLY

Steam holds benefits for almost all skin types, but there are some conditions that it can exacerbate. If you have severe acne, rosacea or a dry skin condition like eczema or psoriasis, seek medical advice before you try steaming. Avoid altogether if you're using products like retinol, which cause the skin to peel.

249 GO DRY

If your skin suffers from dullness and breakouts, a sauna could be a great way to clear those pores and encourage detoxification. Aim to stay in the dry heat for around 15 minutes, subject to the usual medical advice, and consider a niacin supplement to further boost detoxification.

250 PROTECT YOUR SKIN

Saunas act as a workout for the skin's stratum corneum layer so it stays more hydrated. Aim to use one once or twice a week, preferably after exercising, and take a shower afterwards.

251 GET BOOSTED

Inside a sauna your pulse rate can increase by as much as a third, and skin temperature rises to around 40°C (104°F), allowing twice as much blood to flow to the skin as usual, which means the tissues are left oxygenated and vital, with a rosy glow for many hours afterwards. Be careful if you are on medication or have an underlying condition; always seek medical advice first.

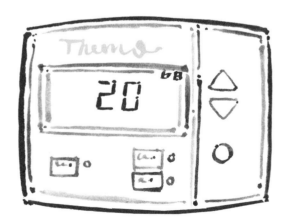

252 CLEANSE FIRST

Because the heat from a sauna causes skin to sweat, flushing out toxins, it's important that the skin is thoroughly cleansed (and preferably also exfoliated) before you go inside. If skin is dirty or blocked with make-up, dead skin or other creams and oils, the health benefits will be far fewer.

253 GET ANTI-BACTERIAL

Saunas cause an increase in sweating, which is thought to benefit the skin because sweat contains an anti-bacterial substance called dermicidin believed to help repel bacteria. But be careful to guard yourself against infection from the sauna too – always use a clean towel, try to avoid touching others and shower afterwards.

254 GO COLD

Showering in cold or lukewarm water after your sauna is thought to benefit the skin by closing up pores, thus preventing infection from entering. If you don't enjoy an ice-cold blast, cool or lukewarm water is perfectly fine.

255 GET CREAMY

Always cleanse and moisturize after a sauna. The skin has been stimulated, so take advantage of all that extra oxygenation by applying creams to help your skin hydrate, tone and stay smooth. Moisturizing is particularly important if you have dry skin.

256 DRINK UP

The reason why saunas are thought to hold such a lot of health benefits is because they encourage your body to sweat more than usual, but this also means water is lost at a much higher rate for several hours afterwards so dehydration can be a danger. Drink up before you start.

257 AVOID ALCOHOL

The night before and the day of your sauna visit, avoid alcohol entirely. It has a dehydrating effect, which, combined with the extra heat of the sauna, can cause the body to overheat. It's best to avoid drinking for 24 hours before exposure to the heat.

258 GET STEAMY

Beauticians often use steam before a salon facial to prepare the skin for treatments because it softens skin, brings dirt and impurities to the surface and allows products to penetrate more easily. Achieve the same benefits at home by steaming for five minutes before your own beauty regime.

259 DON'T GO OVERBOARD

The best way to get steamy benefits for your skin is to keep it regular – whether it's visiting the steam room at a gym or spa, sitting in the sauna or steaming your face at home. Once a week is enough or your skin can start to feel dry and dehydrated.

260 RUB IT IN

After a steam your face is highly receptive to the benefits of products, so indulge in a facial massage with a nourishing oil, such as almond or rosehip. If you have oily or problem skin this is a great time to put on a clarifying clay mask.

261 ADD SOME SCENT

Adding aromatherapy oils to your at-home facial steam is a great way to deliver extra benefits. For dry skin, choose soothing oils such as camomile, jasmine or rose; oily skin needs lavender, rosemary, peppermint, cedarwood or rosewood, while ylang-ylang is great for combination skin. Tea tree and eucalyptus oils suit skin troubled with acne or other problems.

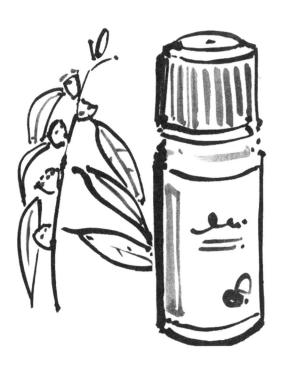

self-facial massage

262 START CLEAN

Before beginning a facial massage, make sure that not only your face but also your hands are cleansed thoroughly. Choose a mask, moisturizer or oil to suit your mood or requirements and find a comfortable position to perform the massage.

263 PAT IT RIGHT

Gently patting the skin under the eyes is a great way to boost blood flow, stimulating regeneration. Remember always to use gentle movements around your eyes – gently pat fingertips around each eye socket in a slow circle.

264 EYES RIGHT

To give your eyes a lift, massage the upper eyelid with your middle finger. Starting at the inside corner of the eye, move just under the eyebrow in small gentle circles towards the temple. Repeat three times.

265 THE EYES HAVE IT

One of the best ways to wake up tired eyes and reduce puffiness is with a gentle eye massage. Massage your usual eye cream under each eye with a gentle touch from your middle and ring fingers, moving from nose to temple and gently pulling up with each stroke. Repeat three times.

266 DO IT DAILY

Self-massage is a great way to help keep the skin smooth, rejuvenated and wrinkle-free. For best results, aim to spend five minutes massaging your face daily, preferably as part of your morning or evening skincare routine. Incorporate massage with a hot-cloth cleanser, or as you apply your morning moisturizer or night cream.

267 GO FOR THE THROAT

Throat skin is often neglected as it's hidden out of sight under the chin but regular massage can help prevent sagging and wrinkles. Use the backs of both hands to stroke upwards from the base of the neck to the chin in one smooth stroke.

268 CLEAR YOUR HEAD

To prevent wrinkles forming on the forehead, use your palms to massage upwards, smoothing out the skin from eyebrow to hairline (be careful not to pull skin – use a gentle touch and plenty of product). Follow with circular fingertip massage, starting in the centre of the forehead above the nose and working upwards and outwards. Now apply gentle pressure to the forehead with all fingers for the count of five and finish with gentle strokes outwards toward the temple and hairline.

269 GET CHEEKY

Your cheeks are probably the one area of your face that will benefit most from self-massage, as there is less blood flow here than other areas of your face. Imagine three lines across your cheeks – one from the chin above the jawline to the ears, another from the lips to the top of the ears and finally, one from the nostrils to the temples. Massage along each of these lines using five to eight circular motions, followed by one long stroke. Repeat three times.

270 LIPPERY WHEN WET

Massaging your lips can help prevent dry skin by stimulating blood flow and boost the formation of new skin layers. Using the tips of four fingers, apply gentle pressure in circular motions upwards and outwards on both lips, finishing with gentle strokes from the centre to outside edge.

271 GO FOR THE PINCH

One of the best ways to massage the chin and jawline is to go for a series of gentle pressure pinches rather than trying to use a circular motion, which can be jerky. Using the thumb and two fingers of each hand, apply gentle pressure to the chin for a count of three, then move along one finger's width and work your way up to your ears.

272 USE YOUR HEAD

Don't forget the skin of your scalp when performing facial massage – the muscles under the hairline can make a real difference to lines on your forehead and the rest of your face. Use your fingertips to gently massage the front half of your scalp.

273 FOLLOW YOUR NOSE

Massaging the skin on your nose can help boost blood flow and prevent clogged pores and fine lines. If your nose is prone to oiliness or blackheads you can perform this massage as part of your hot-cloth cleansing routine or use a facecloth and cleanser. Working upwards from either side of the base of the nose, make small circular movements all the way up to the under-eye area.

facial hair

274 FLATTEN IT OUT

The best tweezers to use for facial hair removal are those with flattened middles and a point for targeting individual hairs, but they are incredibly sharp! Be careful not to dig the ends into your skin, which could cause redness or infection.

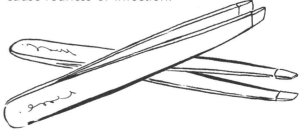

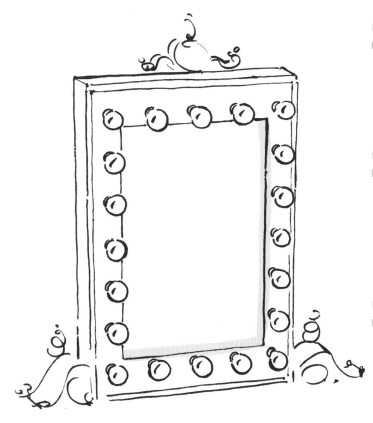

276 BE A NIGHT OWL

When performing your own facial waxing at home, do it last thing at night rather than during the day to give your skin a chance to rest and recover.

277 PARK UP

One of the best places to spot those stray hairs for plucking is a car mirror; it's much lighter in a car than inside most bathrooms. Find a spot where no one will see you and pluck away!

278 TORCH IT

Even under bright light, it's sometimes hard to see what's going on between the ends of your tweezers! Invest in a pair with a light attached between the pincer blades to help illuminate the hair.

275 SHINE A LIGHT

Mirrors with light surrounding them might seem a bit Hollywood but they're a great way to make sure you're removing all your facial hairs. Alternatively, use a desk light targeted on your face.

279 SET THE BOUNDARIES

When using hair removal products such as an epilator at home, set the boundaries first! Use Vaseline to prevent taking off too much hair. Go gently and remove a little at a time instead of large blocks.

280 DON'T BE CAUGHT RED-FACED

If you're visiting a salon for facial waxing or hair removal alongside other treatments, ask for the hair removal to be done first. That way you'll give the skin time to calm down following any reaction and won't have to leave the salon red-faced.

281 GO COLD

A great way to help calm skin down after facial waxing or plucking is to apply an ice pack from the fridge to the affected areas. Use a specially made children's ice pack – these are smooth, small and therefore easy to use on smaller areas such as the upper lip, chin and eyebrows.

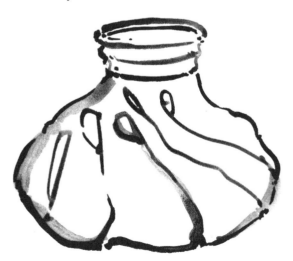

282 MAGNIFY IT

A great way to get a good look at the hairs on your face is with a magnifying mirror but the inside of rooms is often too dark – use it near a window or invest in one with suckers that you can stick to a lit window or mirror for the best view.

lips & eyes

283 BRUSH AND GO

If your lips are seriously dry or flaky, apply a little lip balm. Brush with a soft, dry toothbrush to boost circulation and remove all the dead skin cells while working the moisturizer into the deeper levels of your skin.

284 DON'T LICK YOUR LIPS

Dry, cracked or chapped lips are caused by harsh weather conditions or dehydration. Don't be tempted to lick your lips, though – this only makes them dryer. Have a drink of water and use a lip balm or moisturizer to restore plumpness instead.

285 CHOOSE CAREFULLY

Some common ingredients in lip balm can actually make lips feel dryer. For example, mineral oil (petroleum jelly) creates a film on lips that can signal some skins to halt production of moisturizing lipids; strong flavours and colours also make lips dry. Seek out naturally "breathable" balms such as shea and cocoa butter and beeswax.

286 CITRUS SMOOTHER

A great way to help your lips appear smooth and free of dry skin is to harness the natural power of fruit acids. Eat one piece of citrus fruit each day and after peeling it gently, rub the inside of the skin over your lips to smooth away dead skin from the surface. Wipe clean with a dampened tissue.

287 BREAK THE HABIT

If you have a habit of biting or tugging on your lips with your teeth, which can lead to chapping and dryness, break it over a period of a few days by keeping your lips covered in lip salve. Choose a flavour that you don't like to remind you when you're about to chew.

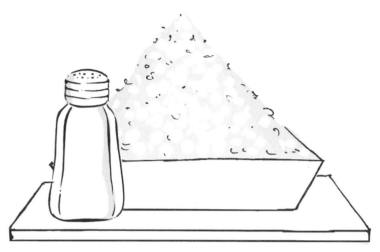

288 SALT YOUR WOUNDS

Rubbing salt onto your lips is a fantastic natural exfoliant. Next time your lips feel dry and flaky, mix up some sea salt with warm water and use on a muslin cloth or face towel to buff lips smooth. Be careful not to swallow, though!

289 MOISTURIZING LIPS

Tackle seriously dry or flaky lips with a lip-facial using a little lip balm. Brush with a soft, dry toothbrush to boost circulation and remove all the dead skin cells while working the moisturizer into the deeper levels of your skin.

280 KEEP TEETH CLEAN

One of the best ways to help the skin on your face appear younger and smoother is to keep your teeth clean. Yellow, cracked teeth can make lips appear dryer too, so make sure you clean your teeth twice a day and apply lip salve or lipstick afterwards.

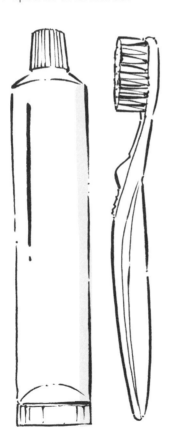

281 HORSING AROUND

Under-eye bags? Creams containing vitamin K and horse chestnut are thought to exert beneficial effects by reducing puffiness and blood flow under the thin skin of the area.

282 KEEP IT LOW

Don't put eye cream on your upper lids before bedtime or you'll wake up with puffy lids. The cream prevents the delicate skin in this area from breathing.

283 GET ELECTRIC

Salon treatments for reducing the wrinkles around eyes include electric therapies, which increase muscle tone by passing a small electric current through the skin, stimulating muscle tone and so reducing wrinkles and fine lines.

284 HAVE AN EXTRA PILLOW

Using an extra pillow can help avoid puffy morning eyes by assisting fluid to drain out of the face by angling it downward. If your neck gets sore, move the pillow under your chest or shoulders.

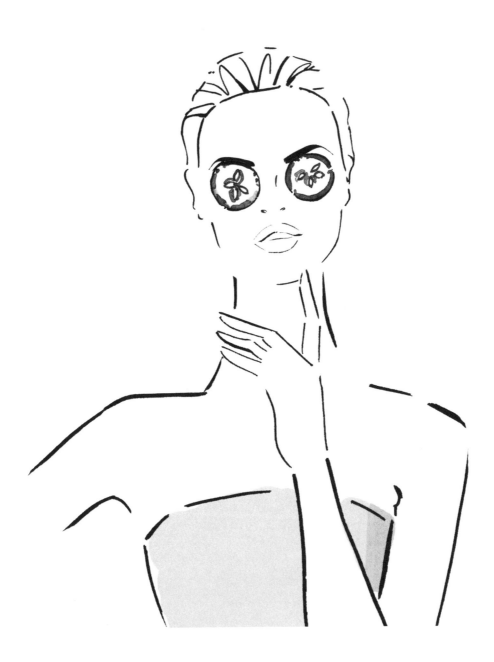

295 CUCUMBER SOOTHER

Place a slice of cucumber on each eyelid for 10 to 15 minutes to allow the high water and mineral content to be absorbed into your delicate eye skin.

296 GO GENTLY INTO THE NIGHT

When you apply night cream under your eyes, do so gently so as not to pull and stretch the skin. Use your fourth finger (which is the weakest) and pat the cream back and forth under the eye, starting at the outer corner and working inward.

297 WAKE UP WITH AYURVEDA

To keep your peepers perky with an Ayurvedic remedy, sprinkle cold water 10 times over tired eyes (keeping them open), morning and night. If you wear contact lenses, do this before you put them in!

298 DE-PUFF WITH ARNICA

Most people know that arnica is a great natural choice for reducing redness, bruising and swelling on minor injuries, but did you also know it can be used to reduce fine lines and puffiness around the eyes, particularly when they're due to tiredness, overwork or illness?

299 MELT THE MELIA

Melia are little pools of oil that form around the eyes, often exacerbated by heavy creams or moisturizers. Beauty salons can offer hot needle treatments to melt the oil away and remove these marks.

300 TRY CRYOTHERAPY

Steal a salon secret for your own home: after applying an eye treatment, place an ice cube inside a small plastic bag, or wrap in clean cotton/muslin. Gently rub over the face and eye area for several minutes to plump up and tone the skin.

exfoliating

301 GET PUFFY

A body puff is one of the best ways to exfoliate your body as you can reach all those hard-to-get areas more easily than with gloves. Also, it feels luxurious and you'll use far less product than with soap or body wash alone. If you want a firmer texture, try a loofah or bristle brush.

302 GENTLY DOES IT

Overly vigorous exfoliating can break the tiny blood vessels under your skin, causing thread veins and redness to appear, especially on the delicate areas around the cheeks, eyes and neck. Be gentle and avoid exfoliators containing natural grains, which tend to be more abrasive than synthetics.

303 FACE FACTS WEEKLY

Once a week, exfoliate your face to remove dead skin cells. This not only makes your skin look fresher and more radiant but also helps products penetrate more deeply into the epidermis, making them more effective.

304 MOISTURIZE ALL THE WAY

If you exfoliate regularly, you should always use moisturizer on your face because the regular exfoliation could lead to skin drying up more easily as a result of having fewer layers. For best results, use it even on the days when you're not exfoliating.

305 STAY NATURAL WITH SALT

Salt is nature's own favourite exfoliant. Not only do the grains help you exfoliate skin gently and without trauma, the natural healing and antiseptic qualities help your skin stay smooth, supple and problem free. But allow it to dissolve a little first to soften the sharp edges.

306 VOTE VOLCANIC

Did you know that some exfoliating cleansers contain as much as 25 per cent ground volcanic rock? These are great for oily skin because they dry up oil without stripping too much out of the skin and causing a rebound effect.

307 TAKE CARE

Don't be tempted to rub too hard or use a too-grainy exfoliant on your face. Instead choose fine-grained products or fabrics and keep it to once a week. If your skin looks red or patchy, you've gone too far.

308 BOTTOM LINE

It might not be the first thing people notice about you, but don't neglect the skin on your buttocks, which can be prone to pimples and cellulite, if left unattended. Use a bath mitt or puff to gently exfoliate in the bath or shower.

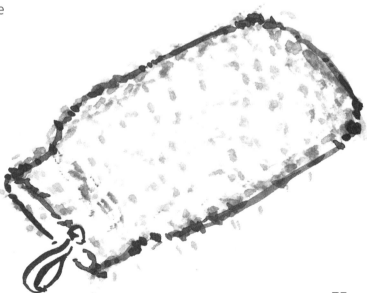

309 MAKE YOUR OWN

For a super-smoothing skin exfoliant, massage a handful of Epsom salts with a tablespoon of olive oil over wet skin. This will cleanse, exfoliate and soften any rough spots. Rinse off well for a polished finish.

310 BE AVOCADO FAIR

Avocado is another natural exfoliant. Finely grate an avocado stone with a small grater and add to a little yogurt, cream or avocado flesh. Use the mixture to polish the skin, then rinse off.

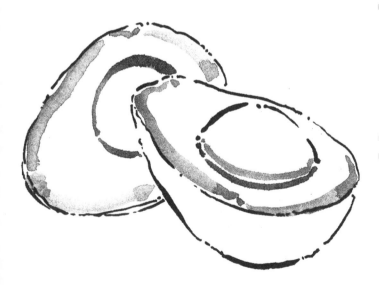

311 TINGLE AWAY

In general, if your skin tingles after exfoliation, this means you've used too harsh a product. However, it is natural to experience a light tingle for up to 15 minutes after using alpha- or beta-hydroxy acids because of their intended chemical effect.

312 SHIELD IN THE SUN

Newly exfoliated skin is more prone to sun damage, so apply sun block after exfoliating if you're heading for the beach.

313 RUB AWAY ROUGH ELBOWS

If your elbows are very dry, put a small amount of foot exfoliator in the palm of your hand and rub in circular motions. This will be too harsh for the skin on your arms, but works a treat on elbows.

314 AVOID MIXING IT

Don't be tempted to use body exfoliators on facial skin because products designed for the body are likely to be harsher and could be too abrasive for your face, resulting in irritation and broken veins.

315 EXFOLIATE BUMPS

It's not just your face that needs exfoliating – skin bumps on legs can occur as a result of ingrown hairs. To avoid them, exfoliate legs regularly with a grainy scrub in the shower or a body puff before applying moisturizer.

scrubs & polishes

316 KEEP IT REGULAR

Your scrub will only keep for a few weeks before it starts to go off, even if stored in an airtight container in a cool place, which maximizes shelf life. For a long-lasting formula, make sure that it contains a natural preservative like rosemary oil extract or grapefruit seed extract.

317 SUPER SALTS

Scrub recipes will call for salts but there are many different types that you can use. Most experts agree that Dead Sea salts are the most therapeutic, followed by natural rock or sea salt and then table salt.

318 CHOOSE YOUR GRAIN

Home-made scrubs and polishes are produced from a choice of three basic ingredients, which have exfoliating properties: salt, sugar or oatmeal. Of these, sugar is the most grainy, followed by salt, then oatmeal, which is much milder, so choose your scrub accordingly.

319 STORE IT WELL

When making up your own scrubs, it makes sense to do so in bulk but always make sure that your storage is up to scratch so that you can avoid bacteria growing and reducing the effects. Always mix and store ingredients in clean glass bowls and jars to prevent any reaction – wash everything in the dishwasher set to at least 65°C (150°F) to kill germs.

320 GO MILD

Oatmeal is a milder option for sensitive or inflamed skin. Combine with yogurt for a double-soothing effect; you can also add honey to help bind the oatmeal together and maximize the exfoliating benefits.

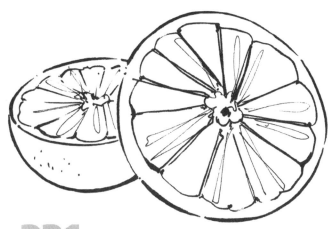

321 GO HERBAL

For a refreshing morning herbal scrub, mix together half a cup of brown sugar, a quarter of a cup of almond oil and five drops each of lavender and peppermint essential oils. Or go citrus by substituting grapefruit, orange, lemon or bergamot oil. For added zing, include lemon or grapefruit zest.

322 SMOOTH DREAMS

A great evening exfoliator to help you sleep with smooth skin is a lavender sea salt scrub. Mix together equal amounts of fine sea salt and olive oil, then add six drops of lavender essential oil or a few handfuls of fresh lavender flowers for a calming scent.

323 GET SWEET

A great choice for a relaxing evening scrub is vanilla and brown sugar mixed with almond or olive oil, which is a great way to help you unwind. Add a few drops of lavender, clary sage or rose oil to make it even more luxurious.

324 CAFFEINE KICK

Coffee grounds are another good choice for exfoliating and they have long been thought to help reduce cellulite when used as part of a scrub. Mix together coffee grounds (used ones are fine as they are already damp) with brown sugar. Add some honey and almond or jojoba oil to bind the ingredients together.

325 SEA-SALT SCRUB

A great exfoliating scrub for general day-to-day use on all skin types is a sea salt scrub (fine sea salt is best because others can be too sharp-edged) with a cup of fine sea salt and half a cup of oatmeal, mixed together with extra virgin olive oil and a few drops of geranium oil. Use twice a week to keep skin buffed and beautiful.

natural bodycare

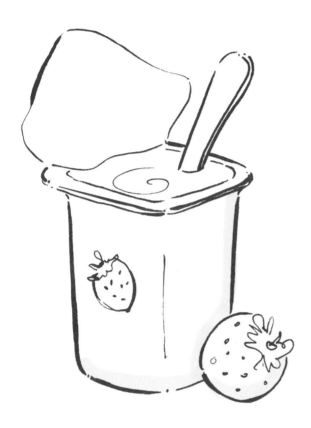

327 BRUSH UP ON SKINCARE

The skin is designed to eliminate toxins and body brushing is thought to help by stimulating circulation and lymphatic drainage. Starting at the feet, brush toward the heart in long, firm strokes without scratching or pulling the skin. Sensitive skin? Wet your brush first to decrease friction, so lowering the chance of adverse reactions. Or try oil instead, but don't brush sensitive skin more than once a week.

328 WAX AWAY CRACKS

Wax is a great overnight treatment to help repair dry areas on feet and damaged and cracked heels. To stimulate skin healing, heat some candle wax up with mustard oil until it melts. Leave until warm before applying to heels and other dry areas. Wear loose cotton socks to bed and wash off in the morning. Note: if heels are cracked and sore and nothing seems to work, you may be suffering from Athlete's foot. If in doubt, seek medical advice.

326 SUPER SOFTENER

For a really gentle exfoliant, combine lactic-acid-rich natural yogurt with fine-grained white sugar and some light olive oil, almond oil or baby oil. Rub into the skin gently with long, soft strokes.

329 CITRUS BRIGHT

Lime and lemon juice contain acids that can help lighten skin patches. Rub the juice over knees and elbows and leave for 15 minutes before rubbing with damp hot flannels or towels. Repeat daily until you see results (one to two weeks). If your skin is cracked, mix the juice with coconut or almond oil to avoid stinging.

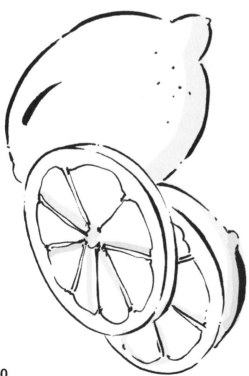

330 USE NORMAL SOAP

Normal soap is almost as effective as anti-bacterial soap for getting rid of germs because most antibacterial soaps must be left on the skin for several minutes before they take action. Besides, many common illnesses are due to viruses, which are not affected and antibacterial ingredients can also cause dehydration.

331 HEAL YOUR HEELS

If your heels are cracked and dry, the juice of an onion can help repair some of the damage. Lightly roast an onion and liquidize or mash to make a paste. Smooth onto heels and leave for 15 minutes before washing off. Repeat daily for several weeks.

332 HAND ME DOWN

If the skin on your hands is rough and dry you should exfoliate before you apply hand cream or the dead skin will block the cream from working. For a mini-scrub, combine a teaspoon of sugar and a teaspoonful of oil; rub over hands and leave for 10 minutes. Rinse off and apply hand cream.

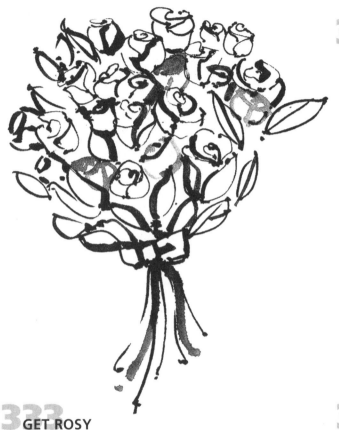

334 WAX LYRICAL

Paraffin wax has long been used as a hand treatment. Melt some paraffin wax with a bit of oil and some essential oils then wait until the wax has cooled enough that a skin forms on top. Test on your wrist to make sure the wax won't burn you. Now wash your hands, coat with olive or coconut oil and dip each one in wax several times. Wait for the first layer to dry before dipping again then put your hands in plastic bags. Rest for 20 minutes before removing the bags and peeling the wax off.

cellulite

333 GET ROSY

Rose is a great choice for calming and nourishing skin. Make up a paste using flour or cornflour mixed with rosewater, then blend together with half a cup each of rose petals (fresh or dried) and milk. Smooth the paste onto your skin and rinse off after five minutes.

335 LIVE WELL

It's widely accepted that avoiding cellulite altogether or getting rid of it altogether is unlikely, but several factors are known to make the appearance worse. These are: yo-yo dieting, living an inactive lifestyle, dehydration or fluid retention, increase in body fat and stress.

336 GRAB SOME GROUNDS

Caffeine has long been used to help those with cellulite improve the appearance of their skin and although the science is inconclusive, many still swear by its skin-stimulating properties. Get your dose by choosing caffeine creams or use coffee grounds (not decaffeinated) in the shower as a scrub.

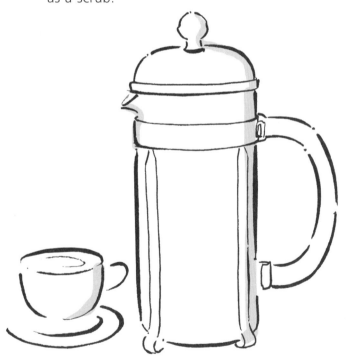

337 GET THE WEIGHT OFF

Losing weight may not get rid of your cellulite entirely, but it will make it appear less obvious and almost certainly reduce the size of affected areas. If you have lots of weight to lose, however, be prepared for things to get worse before they get better as fat disappears from beneath stretched skin.

338 CHOOSE LPG

LPG Endermologie is a salon-based treatment that claims to reduce cellulite through cell stimulation. Painless and noninvasive, it has been found to promote smoother skin after several sessions.

339 TAKE CARE WITH TANNING

Tanning actually makes cellulite look better in the short term because it evens out skin colour to make it less noticeable, but beware when the tan fades! UV light damages the skin, making it thinner and less resilient to stretching, which actually makes cellulite appear worse.

340 REACH FOR RETINOL

In some studies, retinol creams of around 0.3 per cent potency have been shown to reduce the appearance of cellulite in some people because retinol is thought to stimulate skin tissues, thus creating a thicker top layer of skin, which covers the bumps more effectively.

341 BRUSH IT OFF

Using a firm body brush to stimulate blood flow to the skin can help reduce areas of cellulite by encouraging the skin's natural processes – cellulite often appears in the fattest areas of the body, which have fewer blood vessels. Always brush in long, clear strokes toward the heart and avoid pushing too hard.

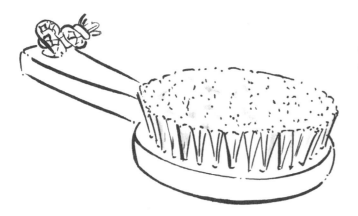

342 CUT THE CREAM

Most anti-cellulite creams make major claims without too much serious scientific research to back them up. Before spending your hard-earned money, check the ingredients list and look for genuine evidence (not before and after photos on the Internet) of its effectiveness. If in doubt, ask a dermatologist.

343 LIKE LIPO

Lipomassage machines use a combination of massage pressure and suction to knead and work the skin, the theory being that they break down the tethered pockets of fat causing the characteristic bumpy appearance of cellulite. Regular treatments are necessary, though, as the skin often bounces back afterwards.

344 IT'S A WRAP

Although there's no evidence that body wraps with bandages actually work to reduce cellulite, the massage beforehand may play a role in cellulite reduction by stimulating blood flow and thus encouraging skin to regenerate.

345 USE A ROLLER

Foam rollers are often used for stretching muscles post-exercise and for targeting injuries or problem areas, but they're also a great anti-cellulite treatment. Simply roll the affected area once or twice a day to help stimulate blood flow and break up fat pockets.

346 GIN SOAK

To a warm bath add a few drops each of the following oils: grapefruit, geranium, fennel, thyme and lavender, then add a shot of gin. Soak for 10 minutes then use a loofah or body brush to massage over your cellulite in upward strokes (toward the heart) for 20 minutes. Afterwards, shower off with a cold blast.

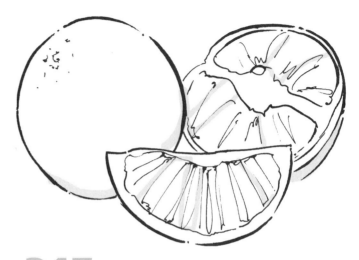

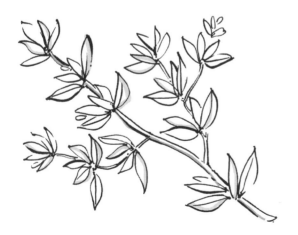

347 REMOVE ORANGE PEEL SKIN

Oranges are a great way to reduce cellulite because of their high water content, which helps to plump skin. Other fruits containing high levels of water are also useful – try apples, grapefruit and tropical fruits such as mango and pineapple.

348 WALKING AWAY

Walking is the best way to reduce cellulite as it tones up the muscles of the legs, hips and bottom and keeps the heart rate gently elevated for fat reduction. For best results, aim for at least 20 minutes, three or four times a week of brisk walking.

349 READY-SALTED

Bathing in salt is thought to reduce cellulite, especially if you add to the benefits by using the grains to give yourself a massage and exfoliation at the same time. Sea salt contains the best balance of minerals, and if you can find Dead Sea salts, they're the best of all.

350 VISIT THE VELA-DROME

Velashape is an anti-cellulite treatment that combines radio frequency with infrared light to target the skin's deeper layers and help rebuild collagen to smooth out skin. If you are younger, a thermal device might work better but it's not suitable for older skins.

351 TUNE IN TO MASSAGE

One salon treatment thought to reduce cellulite, at least in the short term, is the radio massage tool, which delivers heat combined with tissue massage to help break down the connective tissue and fat under the skin. This in turn encourages skin tightening and smooths out surface bumps. The same is true for laser treatments, which have shown at least some temporary benefits.

arms & legs

352 GIVE NATURE A HAND

Every 24 hours, we lose an astounding 10 billion cells from the skin's surface, most of which is on your arms and legs, but it's often a neglected area. Exfoliating once a week or more helps boost this process and prevents pimples and dull skin caused by build-up.

353 CHECK YOUR OIL

If the skin on your face is oily and prone to breakouts, chances are your body has a similar skin type and will benefit from regular exfoliation to avoid dead skin building up and blocking pores, leading to rough skin and spots. Aim to body scrub twice a week, concentrating on the upper arms, legs, bottom and chest.

354 GET BUFF ARMS

If your upper arms are covered in a series of rough red bumps, don't despair! It's likely to be due to a condition called keratosis pilaris, and it's dramatically improved with exfoliation and moisturizing twice a week.

355 STEP IT UP

There's no better way to achieve shapely calves and tighten the skin of lower legs than walking up and downstairs. Ban elevators and escalators for a month and you'll see visible differences.

356 EXFOLIATE BUMPS

It's not just your face that needs exfoliating – skin bumps on legs can occur as a result of ingrown hairs. To avoid them, exfoliate regularly with a grainy scrub in the shower, then apply moisturizer.

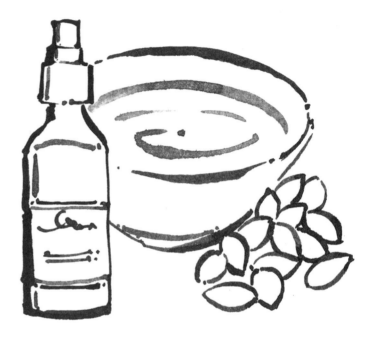

357 HOLD 'EM HIGH

To improve the skin and tone of your lower legs, try to rest your feet above your head for at least 10 minutes a day. This encourages good circulation and blood flow. Lie on the floor with your feet on a chair, or stretch out on the sofa with your feet propped up on the arm while watching television. You could even sneak a nap on the bed with your feet propped up by a couple of pillows.

358 ARM YOURSELF WITH SMOOTHNESS

Slough away rough skin and pimples on arms with regular massage using almond or olive oil to boost circulation. Concentrate on the backs of arms, where fat deposits can cause uneven skin.

359 CIRCLE IT UP

Always apply your moisturizer or body scrub in a circular motion from the ankle up as this boosts the circulation of the blood in the legs, facilitating lymphatic drainage and boosting circulation and, therefore, skin health.

360 STAY MOISTURIZED

If the skin on your lower legs suffers from dryness and flaking, provide a constant boost of moisture by putting on a pair of the latest moisturizing tights. New technology embeds moisturizing agents into the fabric to slow-release throughout the day. It's effective for three to four washes so wear them well!

361 COLD WATER JET

Finish your shower with a jet of cold water aimed at your lower legs. This will stimulate circulation, which can often be sluggish in that area, and also help constrict the blood vessels, thereby boosting the appearance of your legs.

362 MOISTURIZE, MOISTURIZE

Leg skin is particularly prone to dryness owing to hair removal and because our legs are frequently exposed to the elements. Pay them attention by moisturizing them after every bath or shower.

363 CAFFEINE TRIP

Invest in a pair of tights with added caffeine. The idea is that the temperature causes the release of caffeine microcapsules into the skin, so increasing metabolic rate and burning fat to reduce cellulite.

364 GET SMOOTH

For an instant lift, de-fuzz. Smooth legs look shapelier than hairy ones because the hair can reduce skin lines and make them look bigger, especially from a distance. Wax, shave or use a cream regularly.

365 SITTING TARGET

Sleeping in a sitting position with your feet on the ground is stressful for the circulatory system and can lead to puffy ankles and reduced blood flow in the legs. Raise legs if you nap on an armchair or lie down to give circulation a boost.

neck & décolleté

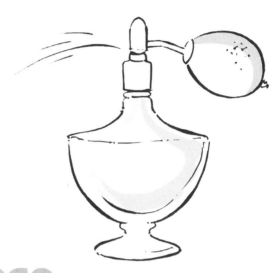

366 MINIMIZE NECK DAMAGE

Don't neglect to nourish your neck with a rich emollient night cream every evening before bedtime. Often the area from the collarbone up to the jawline becomes prematurely wrinkled because the skin here is thinner and more vulnerable than on your face.

367 CARE FOR YOUR CLEAVAGE

When applying day or night cream always remember to include your chest area, from the top of your bust to your neck. Without extra moisturizer the skin here becomes thin and crêpe-like, which can be a telltale sign of ageing.

368 BUST-FIRMER

The Ionithermie bust-firming treatment uses a combination of thermal clay and algae that is spread all over the chest. Two types of electric current are then alternated through this layer, to tone and support the muscles around the breast area, visibly lifting the bust.

369 DITCH THE PERFUME

If you suffer from problem skin, spots or rashes on your neck, consider abandoning your daily spritz of perfume because the alcohol it contains can cause adverse reactions in skin. Apply to wrists and dot behind the ears instead.

370 FERULIC ACID FOR PHOTODAMAGE

The décolleté is prone to photoageing, so protect it with a serum containing ferulic acid (a natural antioxidant produced by most plants). It's particularly beneficial for skin suffering redness (erythema) or which is photodamaged or hyperpigmented.

371 BREAST IS BEST

Improve your bust line simply by standing up straighter. Good posture naturally lifts the ribcage, enabling the breasts to sit more upright on the chest. Imagine a golden string pulling your head upwards right through your crown and try to take your weight in the bottom part of your abdomen, just above your pelvis.

372 CHOOSE IDEBENONE

Look for skin-firming creams and serums specially formulated for the neck and décolletage areas, especially those containing idebenone, a potent antioxidant claimed to alter the reaction of free radical damage and protect skin lipids.

373 INSTANT UPLIFTER

Although there is little apart from surgery that you can do to lift a sagging bosom, you can improve skin texture and tone, and temporarily firm the skin by using a serum specially formulated for this area. Skin will look less slack and appear tighter, but the effect only lasts a few weeks.

374 OPEN YOUR TREASURE CHEST

One really effective treatment to help reduce wrinkles and sagginess on the décolleté is a salon technique known as "derma-rolling". Sharp, extremely thin pins attached to a roller prick through to lower skin levels and encourage healing and wrinkle removal, so it's a great choice for chest skin.

hands & feet

375 QUICK CHECK

Nails are an extension of the skin on your hands, and they're a great way to tell if something is going wrong inside your body. Study your nails carefully every week or two to give yourself a quick self-diagnosis.

376 GET SOME WRIST ACTION

To ease tired hands and give yourself a circulation boost, hold both hands in front of you, palms facing inwards. Loosen their wrist grip and flap backwards and forwards. Feel them tingle as the blood rushes to them.

377 GET SCENTED

Hand cream is a great way to carry your favourite fragrance around with you. If you feel in need of a boost, simply rub some cream into your hands, put them close to your face and breathe deeply. As well as keeping the skin on your hands supply, it will help you take a micro-moment out.

378 SOAK UP SOME MOISTURE

For hands that are smooth and wrinkle-free, soak in a bowl of warm water for five minutes before drying and adding your favourite hand cream. The water soaks into the skin and the cream forms a barrier, locking it in and easing aches and pains at the same time.

379 MINTY-FRESH

Peppermint is cooling and soothing, which means it's the perfect choice for foot treatments. Make yourself up a foot scrub with two cups of sea salt to one cup of olive oil and peppermint essential oil. Massage all over the feet to help remove dry skin and encourage circulation.

380 STRENGTHEN WITH SULPHUR

One of the best supplements for skin, hair and nail health has been shown to be MSM, a special form of sulphur that strengthens the structure of skin. A daily or weekly supplement is a great way to ensure your skin has the strength it needs.

381 434 HONEY HEALER

Honey is a natural moisturizer and you can use it to help heal cracked and chapped feet, especially in winter. Add some to a footbath or mix with half a cup of warm water and paint onto feet. Relax for 20 minutes before rinsing off.

382 HEEL THYSELF

A great tip for preventing build-up of dry skin on heels is when applying daily moisturizer to your legs continue the cream down past your ankle and under your heel. The cream works as a barrier to dry skin formation and prevents you having to use a dedicated foot cream. Be sure your heels are smooth before you begin, though.

383 SCRUB 'EM SMOOTH

Make up a home-made hand exfoliator scrub using almond oil and brown sugar mixed together with some chopped rosemary and lavender flowers. "Wash" onto hands for 10 minutes taking care to massage the backs of hands and the sides of the fingers as well as the palms. Rinse and apply hand cream.

384 SWELL TIME

If you find your feet start to swell after too much time on your feet (especially in vertiginous heels), give them a five-minute booster. Lie with your feet elevated above your head, circling your ankles for a fluid-relieving boost.

385 SOFTLY, SOFTLY

When pumicing your feet, stop if it starts to hurt – you may be taking off too many layers of skin, which can actually cause skin to produce more protective hard layers as a result. For best results, use soft strokes and regular treatments.

386 TREAT WHILE YOU SLEEP

For an overnight treatment for cracked heels, massage a tablespoon of olive oil mixed with a few drops of lemon juice into heels and other dry areas on your feet. Wear cotton socks to bed, then rinse well in the morning and pat dry.

387 GET YOUR ROCKS OFF

A clever way to multitask your feet while enjoying a foot soak is to add some smooth marbles, rocks or pebbles to the bottom of your bowl or bath. This gently stimulates circulation as you soak.

stomach & back

388 GO FOR THE BURN

The best way to tone abdominal muscles is to make sure you exercise them until they fatigue (but you should never feel the strain in your back or hips). The skin will benefit from multiple small repetitions followed by a couple of longer, slow versions.

389 ALL-ROUNDER

If you're scrubbing your stomach to exfoliate, do it in large circles, starting from the right hip and moving upwards, over to the left and round above your pelvis. This follows the line of your large intestine, boosting digestion too.

390 BEAR-LIKE RUB

One way to exfoliate and stimulate circulation in the skin of your back is to lie on a towel on the floor (or lean against it on a towel rail) and rub your back against it just as a bear would against a tree. Do this after your bath or shower.

391 PINCH TO TONE

To tone up a flabby abdomen, activate circulation in the flesh on your tummy with large pinching movements (use your whole hand, not just fingertips) and circular massage. Finish off by briskly rubbing with oiled hands.

392 BACK SCRATCHER

Using a long-handled body brush or loofah is a great way to exfoliate the skin on your back as it enables you to reach hard-to-tackle areas – since it's some of the thickest skin on the body, it can usually withstand the extra pressure. If that feels too scratchy, cover the end of the brush or loofah in a towel or facecloth.

393 REACH FOR THE SKY

One of the best exercises you can do to tone your stomach skin is to reach upwards with your hands. "Grab" the air from above, above right and above left of you, then pull it back towards your stomach.

salon treatments

394 LASER VEIN REMOVAL

Laser energy is absorbed by the blood in the veins to create heat, which damages the lining of the blood vessel, causing the walls to stick together and seal themselves off. The vein is then gradually absorbed by the body and completely disappears.

395 FLOAT ON

However nice your bathroom might be, your bath is just too small for a true flotation experience! Excellent for toning and relaxing, flotation takes away gravity for a while and helps your body and mind relax in peace.

396 HOT SUGAR BODY POLISH

Don't try this one at home, unless you're prepared to caramelize yourself! Hot sugar solution is applied to the skin and all-over massage used to stimulate circulation and boost skin glow. Not only does it exfoliate and rehydrate skin, the massage boosts circulation too.

397 DARTH VASER

VASER (Vibration Amplification of Sound Energy at Resonance) is a form of ultrasound-assisted liposuction, which uses sound waves to break down fat before extracting it from different areas of the body. Although invasive, it is less damaging than traditional liposuction as it causes less trauma to the surrounding skin.

398 DEAD SEA TREATMENTS

You can also do these at home (see page 215), but the more powerful ingredients are reserved for salon formulations. With their plentiful minerals, Dead Sea treatments help detoxify and revitalize skin.

399 BE A JEWEL

Some problem skin can respond to electronic gem therapy, which involves passing light rays through gemstones. For eczema sufferers, emeralds and sapphires are used to zap problem areas.

400 BODY SCULPTOR

Thalgo's "Slim and Sculpt" treatment is designed to specifically target fatty deposits and help the body to break them down by improving circulation and lymphatic drainage, as well as stimulating muscle activity.

body wraps & massage treatments

401 WRAP AWAY PAIN

Some body wraps are designed to target pain such as muscle soreness and joint problems. Soaking bandages in naturally "healing" products such as arnica can help.

402 GET WEEDY

A seaweed or algae body wrap can help hydrate and smooth skin as well as remove toxins from the surface because the extracts are naturally high in salt and also has a similar structure to skin, which eases the transfer of chemicals. Detoxifying wraps can also boost the immune system.

403 DRINK IT IN

Body wraps are designed to remove water from the skin, which is why it's claimed they reduce toxin levels and create measurable water loss. So it's doubly important to keep hydrated, before and after treatment, drinking 20 per cent more than on a normal day.

404 SWEAT IT OUT

Body wraps are designed to wrap the skin tightly, encouraging detoxification by sweating and drawing out impurities. This treatment is even more powerful if combined with massage, which is known to boost circulation. For best results, enjoy a massage first, followed by a body wrap. Inch loss is temporary, skin health longer lasting!

self-massage

405 MULTITASKING MASSAGE

When applying moisturizer, do so with massage techniques: use sweeping, upward motions toward your heart to give your lymphatic drainage a boost and even out skin tone.

406 BE A TENNIS PRO

Instead of shelling out for an expensive salon massage, make your own back relaxer. Lie on your back with a couple of used tennis balls positioned at the top of your buttocks or lower back. Now roll around to release tension.

407 GET YOUR HAND IN

Give your circulation a mini-boost when you apply hand cream using small, circular movements to rub cream into knuckles and joints. Use thumbs to gently massage the backs of hands.

408 ALMOND OIL UPLIFTER

The thin skin on the breasts is prone to sagging and toxin build-up. Massage problems away using almond oil and gentle sweeping strokes from the underside up into your armpits.

409 DON'T USE A MIRROR

During massage, a mirror can be distracting, especially when concentrating on the facial area. Instead trust your touch instincts and use your fingers where it feels right.

410 TOOL UP

Use wooden self-massage tools while you're in the bath for an added boost. The warm surroundings also help to make massage more effective, especially if you're trying to un-knot tense muscles.

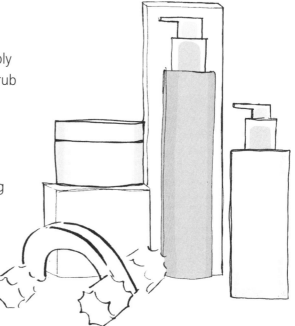

how to use products wisely

411 GO MINIMAL

If you have soft water, you will probably find it takes lots of rinsing to get rid of the product from your face and body. Try using half the amount of product and twice the time rinsing to ensure you don't leave a residue on your skin.

412 SPECIALIZE FOR EYES

For quick and effective action, use a good-quality eye make-up remover rather than a cleanser. The oils it contains will dissolve make-up better and faster than regular cleanser or toner. Afterwards, cleanse as usual.

413 AVOID THE BAD GUYS

Some ingredients in face creams and beauty products actually do your skin more harm than good by stripping away beneficial oils and contributing to inflammatory reactions. Be on the alert for products containing parabens, petroleum, mineral oil, sulphates, phthalates and synthetic dye.

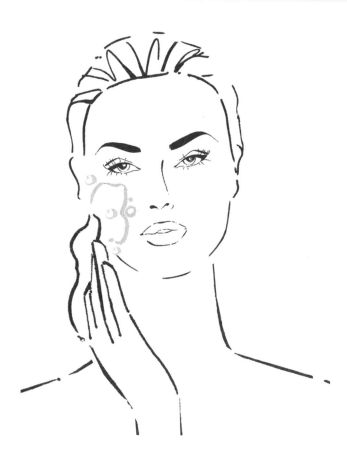

414 GET INTO A LATHER

If it seems you're using a lot of product to create a lather and it washes off super-quick, you probably have hard water. Get into a proper lather by choosing a sulphate-free cleanser.

415 STORE THEM WELL

Beauty products with active ingredients need careful storage to help preserve their life and keep them working effectively. It's no good spending money on an expensive cream then leaving it on a sunny windowsill, near a radiator or even in the car – a cool, dark place is best.

416 OPT FOR ALCOHOL-FREE

If you must use facial wipes for cleansing because you simply haven't got time for anything else, choose an alcohol-free variety because these won't damage your skin. And remember, if you're avoiding alcohol-based cleansers and facial wipes so as not to dry your skin, you should avoid drinking it daily too!

417 CHECK THE USE-BY DATE

Just like the food items in your fridge and cupboard, the ingredients in your skincare products don't last forever. It might seem a waste to throw away something you haven't finished but your skin will thank you. Make sure you throw it away if the consistency, smell or colour has changed too.

looking at labels

418 CHOOSE OILS CAREFULLY

The term "oil-free" was originally used to describe products not containing industrial mineral oil, which were thick and heavy. Nowadays oil-free usually means the product isn't oil-based, which makes them a better choice for acne prone skin.

419 AVOID BLOCKAGES

If you suffer from blackheads, pimples, breakouts or acne, look for the term "non-comedogenic" on the label – it means the ingredients have been tested and shown not to clog up pores.

420 GO HYPO

Many people assume that a product labelled "hypoallergenic" won't cause an allergic reaction, but although it does mean there is less chance of causing a reaction, it doesn't mean no reaction is guaranteed. Look at individual ingredients to check if there's anything you've reacted to before and do a patch test if you're at all unsure.

421 DON'T BE MISLED

Although "dermatologically tested" might sound scientific, there is no standardization for this phrase and others like it, which could mean different things, and they are in no way a sign that the product does as it claims. "Dermatologist recommended" is another vague phrase, as it might only refer to one dermatologist!

422 BE A NATURAL SCEPTIC

There are no specific criteria a product must attain before it can be labelled "natural" – it's often more about the feel. Natural products may contain synthetic ingredients, and truly natural ingredients such as rosemary and lavender can cause reactions in some people too.

423 FILL IN THE BUMPS

Emollients are thicker creams that fill in cracks and rough spots caused by dryness or irritation, making the skin look and feel smoother. Some alcohols, such as cetyl and isostearyl, are emollients, along with sunflower, almond, avocado and coconut oil.

424 ORDER ORGANIC

In some countries of the world, products that use the label "organic" must adhere to strict guidelines on production, chemical use and often the treatment of workers too, but some companies are far more lax. Before you trust the label, check to see what the word "organic" really means – the same goes for "skin organics" and "natural organics".

425 HUM FOR HUMECTANTS

Humectants are products that attract moisture to the upper layers of the skin, making it appear more hydrated and plumper, and flooding it with the right level of moisture to grow and repair effectively. On labels these appear as glycerin, panthenol, ceramides and urea.

426 GET A FILM

Occlusives work by covering the skin with a thin film that prevents moisture from escaping, but they can cause acne and clog pores if used on the wrong skin. Varieties include paraffin, cetyl palmitate, dimethicone and mineral oil.

427 BE BOTANICAL

If you see the word "botanical" on the label of a product, it means that some of the ingredients are derived from plants and/or trees, such as tea tree extract, aloe vera and eucalyptus. But be aware that just because they are plant based, it doesn't mean they won't cause skin reactions.

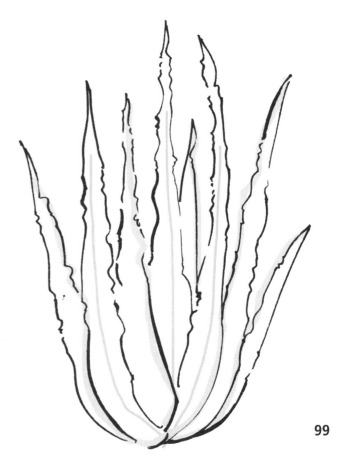

428 SCRATCH THE SURFACE

Surfactants promote lathering and foaming action and make creams easier to apply and use by altering texture. These include ammonium lauryl sulphate, cocamidopropyl betaine and stearates.

429 GO NATURAL

You might not want artificial preservatives in your products, but you do want them to last. T-50 vitamin E oil is a natural antioxidant that helps prevent degeneration to extend shelf life. Look for it on labels as "T-50" or "tocopherol".

430 BE PARABEN-FREE

Parabens are synthetic compounds used as preservatives to prevent bacteria, mould or other microbes ruining the product. Found on labels as methylparaben, ethylparaben, propylparaben and butylparaben, they may cause dryness and irritation.

431 BEWARE THE BADDIES

Not all parabens are labelled as such. Other preservatives derived from parabens are LiquaPar oil, Germaben, Phenonip and Germall.

432 GET IN LINE

The general rule is that ingredients are listed on labels to show that those at the beginning of the list are present in higher concentrations while those at the end are in lower concentrations, except for drugs (listed before other ingredients) and fragrances, dyes and colours (often listed last). Ingredients below 1 per cent concentration can be listed in any order, but they must be after those with higher concentrations and, remember, active ingredients may not need to be in high concentrations to do their work.

433 LOOK FOR THE GOOD GUYS

If a product is labelled "alcohol free" this simply means that it doesn't contain ethyl or SD alcohol, which is typically harsh and dehydrating for the skin (some companies add it to remove oil from the skin). There are some beneficial alcohols, however – cetyl alcohol and stearyl alcohol are emollients from coconut oil used as stabilizers. Cetearyl alcohol is an emulsifying wax and lanolin alcohol, which is the oil extracted from sheep's wool, is used in the same way.

434 SULPHATE ALERT

For many people, products containing sulphates (or sulfates) won't have any effect on the skin, but others find they can cause dryness and irritation. If your skin tends to be reactive and prone to reactions, it's probably worth avoiding them.

435 GRAB A GRAPEFRUIT

Grapefruit Seed Extract (GSE) is an anti-microbial used as a preservative in some skin products, usually in combination with glycerin to keep it stable; it's rare that it causes reactions and is often found on labels as grapefruit extract (*Citrus grandis*).

436 KNOW YOUR NAMES

Vitamins in creams are often given by their generic names rather than listed as "vitamin A" and so on. Look for tocopherol (vitamin E), Retinol (vitamin A), ascorbic acid (vitamin C) and folic acid (vitamin B).

437 REMEMBER ROSEMARY

Rosemary Oil Extract (ROE) is another natural anti-microbial and antioxidant product. It's often found on labels as rosemary leaf extract (*Rosmarinus officinalis*), but remember, it's a powerful product that can cause a reaction in some skins.

438 AVOID ARTIFICIAL

Artificial colours and fragrances do nothing apart from making skincare products smell or look nice. In some cases, though, they can cause sensitivity, breakouts and irritation.

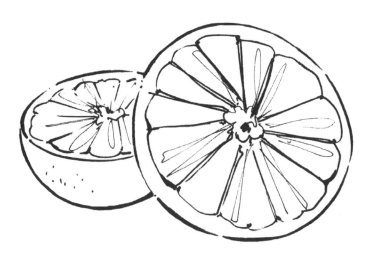

regular & tinted moisturizers

439 AVOID YOUR EYES

Facial moisturizers are not designed for use around eyes – the skin around the eye area is different from the rest of the face, and facial moisturizers can cause oil to be trapped beneath the skin. Stick to an eye cream.

440 GIVE IT A REST

Moisturizer seals in more than moisture – it stops oil escaping from the skin and can cause spots in those prone to breakouts. Give yourself the occasional break from nighttime creams to allow your skin to breathe and regulate normally.

441 LET IT SOAK IN

Moisturizers are not meant to soak into the skin right away, so allow time before leaving the house or applying make-up to get the full effects and avoid streaking.

442 GO EASY ON THE SHIMMER

Many "shimmer" or "light reflective" creams are designed for evening coverage, which means if you wear them in bright sunshine you can light up like an airport runway! Before you leave the house, make sure you check your face in the light you're going to be seen in.

443 COVER UP FIRST

If you want the light, natural application of tinted moisturizer but you have some problem areas to cover up (such as under-eye bags or spots), make sure you apply your cover-up first and choose a creamy product about half a shade lighter than your skin tone. Blend and apply.

444 DO IT DAMP

The best way to apply almost any moisturizer is to leave your skin a little damp after cleansing. It shouldn't be dripping wet, but if you pat dry rather than wipe the towel across it, you'll leave more moisture on the skin.

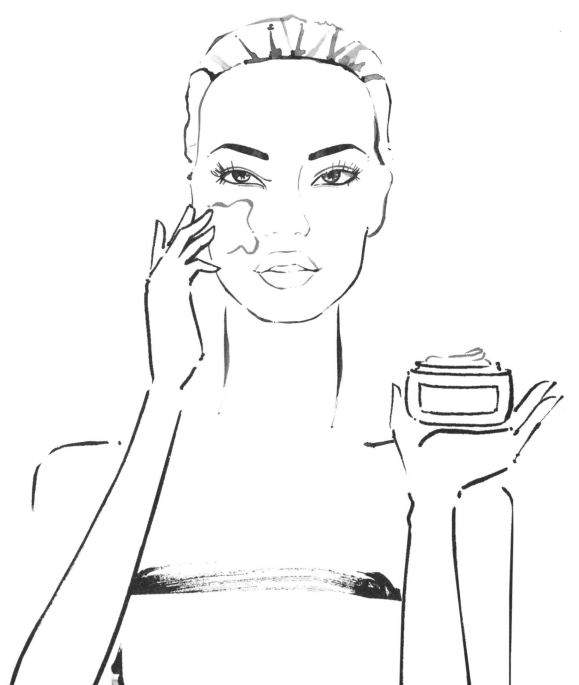

445 DO THE DAYTIME DASH

Tinted moisturizer is really easy to apply and gives a sheer coverage with few application lines, which makes it a great choice if you're dashing out in the morning but don't want to look washed out. Apply over the whole face with fingertips.

446 USE A SPONGE

Put tinted moisturizer on a dry make-up sponge to help it go on more smoothly. Dab onto the forehead and blend up toward the hairline, then the nose, jawline (blending down to neck) and finally, across cheeks.

447 PREPARE YOUR PALATE

Before you apply tinted moisturizer, make sure you prepare your skin for an even application. Cleanse and pat dry, then apply a small amount of moisturizer (you don't want to over-cover skin); allow to soak in thoroughly, then apply.

448 SPRAY IT ON

If you're in a rush first thing, choose a spray-on tinted moisturizer for light coverage and fast application. Cover your clothes first, though, to avoid spraying with product.

449 PALM IT ON

Many people apply far too much product. Put a pea-sized amount in the palm of your hand and rub the palms together to start warming up the moisturizer. Spread over palms, then start with cheeks, the neck, forehead, nose and chin.

450 SLAP ON A SERUM

Serum can make a great make-up base, especially for oily skin, which can suffer if too many layers of moisturizer are applied. Smooth it on after cleansing.

toners & mists

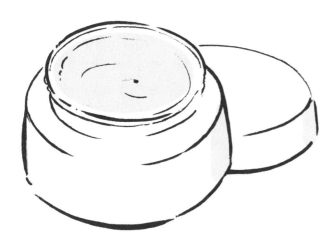

451 KEEP IT LIGHT

Tinted moisturizers are designed for light coverage and don't look good when applied too thickly. It's best to start light with a pea-sized amount and build up the coverage gradually than to begin with too much.

452 MOISTURIZE FIRST

Don't fall into the trap of thinking a tinted moisturizer will do the same job as a moisturizer, as well as cover your skin. Designed to add a sheer wash of colour, it goes on best over your regular moisturizer.

453 TELLING TINGLE

In general, products that cause tingling are too harsh – tingling in response to toners or cleansers is your skin's way of telling you to go for something weaker. Try toners that are designed for sensitive skin – look for those based on rosewater instead of alcohol.

454 POUR COLD WATER ON IT

For a quick tone and boost for tired, dull skin, splash your face in cold water to bring fresh blood to the surface, stimulate circulation and give a healthy glow.

455 GET CITRUS FRESH

Make yourself a refreshing toner, particularly good for cooling down your skin on a hot summer's day. Add a handful each of finely grated lemon peel, grapefruit peel and mint leaves to 300 ml (½ pint) of water. Bring to the boil and leave to cool, then strain. Use to refresh the skin as required. It will keep in the fridge for a few weeks.

456 WITCHES' BREW

If you run out of toner, witch hazel mixed with a little water is a natural alternative but take care with older skins, which can dry excessively if the mix is too concentrated.

457 GET ROSY

If you have combination or dry skin, your toner should be mild and non-astringent to gently boost circulation. Those containing rosewater are a good option.

458 GO-ZONE LAYER

If you have oily skin, or oily areas, consider using a more astringent toner in only those areas. What's good for oily skin can be too harsh for dryer cheeks and foreheads.

459 BE ALCOHOL-FREE

Alcohol-based toners and cleansers are the enemy of dry skin as they strip it dry of moisture and can cause problems with skin firmness and blemishes. If you suffer from dry skin, avoid products with alcohol and use a moisturizer more than once a day to keep skin plump and hydrated.

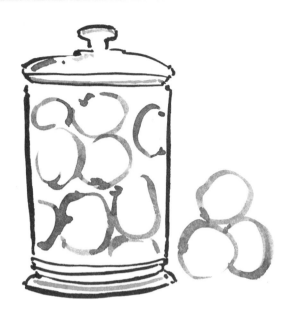

460 HAVE A BALL

Toners are designed to strip oils away from the skin rather than sit on top of it, which is why they're best applied quickly and not rubbed in. Use a cotton-wool ball to wipe smoothly and quickly across the surface of the skin.

461 SPRAY IT ON

If you have sensitive skin, look for a spray toner rather than wipe on, as sensitive skin can become irritated when even a cotton-wool ball is wiped over it.

creams, serums & oils

462 EXTREME CREAMS

Hydroquinone is a common ingredient in skin-bleaching creams, but as it works by killing off the top layers of skin cells, some people find it makes their skin look older and causes sensitivity. Use with care.

463 THINK LONG-TERM

Serums are designed to work on the lower levels of skin, while moisturizers and creams work with the top layers. Using both will give skin a boost in the long- and short-term, so stick to your routine for a few weeks before you judge the results.

464 LESS IS MORE

Avoid slathering on more product than recommended in the belief that it will work better. Many good products are highly concentrated and are designed to be used only in small amounts.

465 BE SENSITIVE

If you have easily reactive or sensitive skin, stick to pure products without a cocktail of anti-ageing or AHA ingredients. These will simply replenish the natural moisture without triggering a problem.

466 USE IT, OR LOSE IT

When applying a face cream, scrub or mask, instead of wiping or washing off what's left, use it up on the backs of hands and fingers to keep them looking younger and well conditioned for longer.

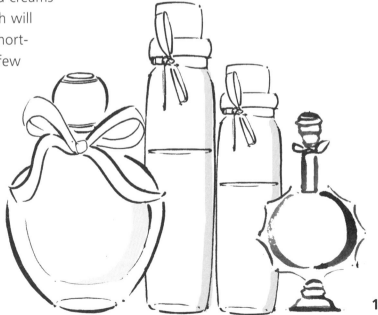

467 GLOW WITH SERUM

Unlike moisturizers, serums – either in bottle form or as ampoules – have an oily rather than absorbent texture and impart a glow to the skin that improves the visual appearance. They can be used as a quick pick-me-up to give an instant richness to skin's texture.

468 MOISTURIZE ONE AT A TIME

It's a common mistake to buy three or four similar products, open them all and use them alternately. If you do this, the chances are that you won't use them all before their use-by date and they'll end up going off and/or becoming ineffective.

miracle ingredients

469 RAM IN THE RHAMNOSE

Rhamnose is a Brazilian plant sugar (also known as cat's claw), which is well known for its soothing properties. Look for it at a 5 per cent concentration to help even out skin tone and colour and reduce pigmentation.

470 B CLEVER

Choose products – especially for use during the day – that contain high levels of B vitamins, and particularly niacinamide. Essential for skin health, this vitamin helps reduce dehydration and boosts collagen and fatty acid levels.

471 HI FOR HYALURONICS

Hyaluronic acid isn't just a great product to help skin to recharge and renew, it's also a good way to get other ingredients into the deeper layers of skin, where they can exert a stronger effect. Look for it in creams and anti-ageing products.

472 GET HELP FROM AHA

Alpha-hydroxy acids (AHAs), which are found in many anti-ageing products, are organic "fruit acids" derived from fruit-bearing plants. They are believed to help generate new collagen, making skin firmer and plumper, and they also dissolve the "glue" that binds dead cells together, allowing them to be washed or cleansed away to reveal younger cells.

473 QUEUE UP FOR CO-Q10

Co-enzyme Q10 is a natural antioxidant found in every cell of the body that helps fight bacteria and free radicals, and allows cells to grow and repair. Incorporated in anti-wrinkle creams, the synthetic version can reduce lines and deter new ones.

474 GO MAD FOR MANGOSTIN

If you suffer from redness, blotchiness and broken capillaries on the skin, look for mangostin in your face cream. An extract from the mangosteen fruit, it has been shown to help reduce red patches, dark spots and other circulation-related troubles, particularly when combined with antioxidant vitamins A, C and E.

475 C THE DIFFERENCE

Vitamin C (ascorbic acid) has a brightening effect on skin as it helps boost circulation and collagen production, which means skin looks and feels firmer and smoother as a result. It is essential to the formation of collagen. Look for it in serums, creams and natural beauty products.

476 GO FOR GLYCERIN

Glycerin is a great choice for skin needing hydration as it "grabs" water toward the skin and prevents it dissolving away, therefore leaving skin feeling supple and hydrated and looking smooth and wrinkle-free. It's especially good in eye creams and anti-ageing formulations.

477 SWING OUT FOR SODIUM

Sodium hyaluronate promotes long-lasting hydration in much the same way as glycerin, and is actually used in keyhole surgery to help increase the viscosity of fluid in knee and shoulder joints. Its main action is to increase elasticity and help cells bind together to make skin feel tighter.

478 REDUCE REDNESS WITH BHAS

BHAs, beta-hydroxy acids that include salicylic acid, help shed excess skin cells with their chemical sloughing effect. They are also anti-inflammatories, which make skin appear less red and inflamed and reduce puffiness. Gentler than AHAs, they can also treat acne.

479 VITAMIN COCKTAILS

BioVityl and VitaNiacin technology is the newest way to give skin a vitamin boost, by combining all the vitamins the skin needs in one formula. The combination of vitamins cleverly increases absorption and makes the creams work better.

480 C FOR YOURSELF

Vitamin C is a natural skin protector, necessary for the formation of collagen. As an antioxidant it destroys harmful free radicals in the body caused by pollution, stress and bad diet. Free radicals attack the skin, causing premature ageing, so vitamin C in creams and diet is a must.

481 ZINC IT UP

When it comes to skin-boosting minerals, zinc is the number one choice as it has a direct effect on the regeneration of skin from the inside out. It not only helps with problem and ageing skins but also gives your skin a healthy glow and banishes dullness.

482 THINK ZINC

Zinc sulphate products such as Cellex-C are naturally derived from plants and sometimes shellfish, and have been claimed to have anti-ageing effects in smoothing the skin and protecting it from dehydration. They can help clear blemish-prone complexions and may improve colour, tone and texture.

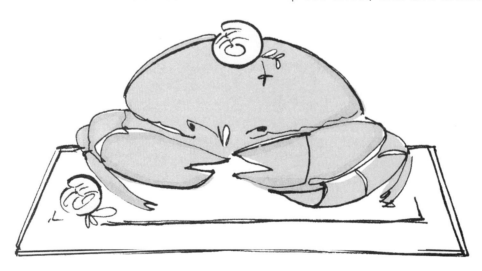

483 REPAIR TISSUES WITH B5

Vitamin B5 is known to assist with tissue repair, which can help the skin to feel smoother and younger because it repairs problems in the deeper layers and prevents blemishes and fine lines.

484 REGENERATE WITH RETINOID

Retinoid is a vitamin A compound, available through pharmacies in the prescription Retin-A and in cosmeceuticals as retinol. It can help reduce fine lines and wrinkles by regenerating skin in the lower layers, sloughing off the upper layers and stimulating collagen and elastin.

485 FADE AWAY FRECKLES

Kojic acid and arbutin are natural alternatives to hydroquinone, which work synergistically to help break up hyperpigmentation in the skin's layers by levelling out melanin levels. They have been used successfully for fading age spots, freckles and sun spots.

486 MAKE MINE A MAGNESIUM

Magnesium has been shown to reduce the appearance of fine lines and wrinkles by helping to tighten the skin surface and boost the production of new skin cells. It is often found as an ingredient in age-defying polishers.

487 LOOK FOR LIPOLIC

Alpha-lipoic acid is nature's most powerful anti-inflammatory and antioxidant treatment, which is many times more powerful than vitamins alone for skin healing and hydration.

488 SAY YES TO SAFFLOWER

Increasingly, cosmetic companies are waking up to the benefits of safflower oil to create and purify emulsions. The product increases the skin's absorption of oils without making it oily, so it's a great choice for anti-ageing creams.

489 LATCH ONTO LACTIC ACID

Lactic acid is a wonderful ingredient for extra moisturization because it helps the skin hold onto the moisture being added through creams and lotions. It's especially useful in anti-wrinkle and anti-ageing products.

490 BOOST OILS NATURALLY

One of the major skin health-boosting ingredients in creams and lotions is essential fatty acids (EFAs), which can plump the skin and help prevent it from drying out with their non-greasy, oil-producing texture.

natural alternatives

491 LOVE CLOVE

Clove oil has antiseptic qualities that can calm the skin, reduce breakouts and blackheads, and smooth away other skin problems. Once used by dentists to help reduce toothache, some people still swear by its anaesthetic qualities.

492 BREATHE DEEP

Eucalyptus oil helps drain away toxins and reduces inflammation; it also acts as a very mild, natural antiseptic. As well as working topically on the skin in face products, it also works to clear sinuses and other membranes, which help reduce puffiness from the inside.

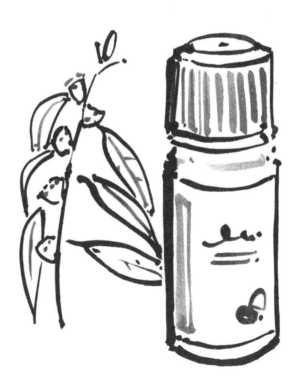

483 BUTTER UP

Cocoa butter is perfect for dry, ageing or damaged skin as it smooths, soothes, reduces inflammation and puffiness, and gives a good dose of antioxidant minerals. It's a great choice for creams because it's rare to find such calming products with high levels of vitamins too.

484 HOP IT

Hops contain high levels of vitamin B complex, which means they deliver a massive antioxidant boost to the skin, but they are also traditionally used to help prevent anxiety and insomnia. They are therefore a great choice for night creams and nighttime products.

485 GO SWISS

Swiss garden cress extract is a relatively new herbal ingredient that has been shown to help even up skin tone and reduce areas of pigmentation and redness in skin surface. It contains high levels of the phytonutrient sulforaphane, which is a powerful antioxidant.

486 CALM WITH CAMOMILE

Camomile is an extremely mild substance that helps soothe away blemishes and skin irritation, softens the skin's surface and aids relaxation. People often drink camomile tea to help them relax and unwind – camomile oil, flowers or as an added ingredient can help do the same for your skin.

487 GO SHEER WITH SHEA

Shea butter is a great natural choice for skincare. Not only is it thought to have anti-inflammatory and humectant properties; it also acts as an emollient to keep skin hydrated. It's also a great choice for day creams as it has some ability to absorb some UV rays.

498 PAPAYA FOR PAPAIN ENZYME

Papaya contains the papain enzyme, a natural, nonabrasive botanical that dissolves dead skin cells, which makes it a great ingredient for face masks and exfoliators. It deep-cleanses without stripping, leaving dull skin smoother and more refined.

499 THYME FOR CUCUMBER

Cucumber contains anti-inflammatory and antiseptic properties to soothe red, irritated skin. It is thought to be especially powerful when used in combination with the garden herb thyme, as the effects are strengthened.

500 GET IN THE GINSENG

Ginseng has long been used as a herbal supplement or tea to help boost energy levels and reduce inflammation in the body, but its main use in skincare is to tone and revitalize skin by boosting blood flow, reducing puffiness and delivering a huge punch of phytonutrients at the same time.

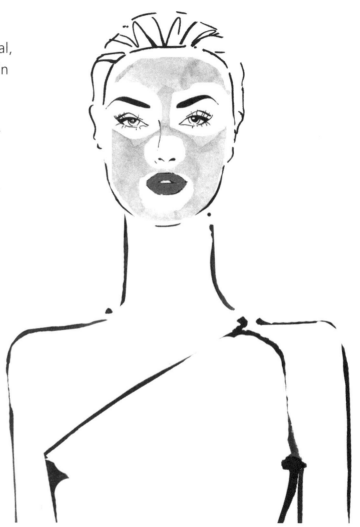

501 GET SMOOTH WITH SOY

Soy proteins can help make skin temporarily smoother by improving firmness and elasticity, if applied regularly. You'll see them listed as ingredients in cutting-edge face creams.

502 EASE ACHES WITH ECHIUM

Echium seed oil is a relatively new addition to the omega-boosting seed oils, containing high levels of omega 3 and 6, but it's a great choice for vegetarian delivery of these essential fatty acids. It's used widely now in skincare because it contains high levels of GLA (Gamma Linolenic Acid) for soothing inflammation and problem skin.

503 RISE WITH ROSE

Rose hip oil is a fantastic choice for facial skincare. Unique among pressed seed oils, it contains naturally high levels of Retinol, as well as vitamin C and essential fatty acids, so it's ideal for skin regeneration. It can also help soothe inflamed skin, remove dried-out top layers and reduce the appearance of fine lines.

504 CRUNCH A CARROT

Carrot oil contains high levels of beta-carotene, which give a good antioxidant boost to skin when included in creams and products. They are also extremely high in flavonoids, which help reduce inflammation and mop up free radicals, reducing skin damage and increasing tone.

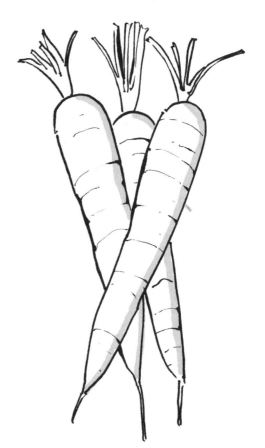

tools of the trade

505 WASH AND BRUSH UP

It's easy to forget that face cloths, sponges, make-up brushes and other beauty tools need cleaning too, or they can become a breeding ground for bacteria that can lead to spots and infection. Make sure you give yours a wash with a specialist cleaner, mild soapy water or mild shampoo once a week and rinse well.

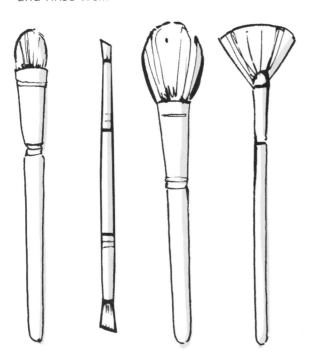

506 DOWN TOOLS

Never use dirty cloths, tools or products on your skin, especially your face. Be smart about product storage (avoid sunlight and warmth) and make sure you don't keep products for longer than their expiry date – if you don't use much, buy smaller packages and replace as soon as they're out of date.

507 DON'T BE A SPONGER

Natural sponges are a great choice for facial skincare as they offer an exfoliant action in the same way as cloths but are naturally resistant to bacteria, so less likely to transfer infection or germs around your skin. For best effect, use small, circular movements.

508 MAKE IT A MUSLIN

Muslin cloths are great for any type of skin – they can be used for cleansing, removing make-up, pressing onto the face to help open pores (with warmth) or to close pores (with cold), gentle exfoliation and revitalizing, They will need to be washed at least weekly, so buying a pack of three is recommended.

508 COTTON RICH

Cotton is one of the latest natural ingredients to hit the headlines, especially in products for dry skins. The structure of cottonseed oils can help skin lock away moisture and stay hydrated for longer.

510 WEAR YOURSELF SLIM

New fabric technology from companies such as Proskins means that not only can wearing tights help you appear slimmer by compression but modern fabrics infused with products such as caffeine, retinol and vitamins actually help reduce cellulite and firm up problem thighs while you wear them.

511 POUND A PUMICE

Foot files are good for very hard skin, but when it comes to keeping your feet smooth and beautiful, there's nothing like a pumice stone used at the end of every bathing session. Don't be tempted to press too hard, if you're using a pumice stone to reduce or get rid of areas of dry skin. Work in small patches, using soft, small motions. To get rid of hairs, rub gently in circular movements.

512 GO CLARISONIC

It might seem like a big investment, but there really is evidence to show that sonic care products like the Clarisonic cleanser do give a deeper clean than other cleansers by removing more product build-up.

513 WEAR GLOVES

One of the best ways to give your skin a quick exfoliating boost is to use exfoliating gloves. Designed to go over your hands, they allow you to lather up your shower cream while rubbing briskly onto skin – you'll receive some massage benefits too.

514 BE FIRM

If you're buying a body brush, choose one that is firm but not scratchy or uncomfortable, either to hold or on your skin as you brush. Detachable long-handled brushes are easier to control than mitts and will reach more areas.

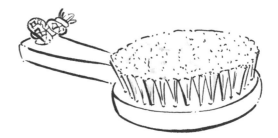

go green

515 HIP TO BE FAIR

Choosing fair-trade goods not only makes certain that the people involved in their manufacture have been fairly treated and rewarded for their labour, it also means the amount of chemicals has been reduced – products are likely to contain far fewer pollutants too.

516 READ THE LABEL

Don't take natural for granted – always read the label. In Europe and the USA, a product can be called "natural" even if only 1 per cent of its ingredients fall into that category. Make sure you're not taken in by these manufacturers' claims.

517 HIT THE BAR

Don't buy soap in plastic bottles, where there is a small amount of soap for a lot of packaging. A greener choice is to opt for soap in bars – these have less packaging and last longer.

518 MIX YOUR OWN OILS

Many bath oils that claim to contain natural products actually contain chemical compounds designed to mimic the smell of herbs and fragrances. Instead of wasting your money on artificial smells, why not mix your own with essential oils?

519 MINIMIZE PACKAGING

Wherever possible and without affecting efficacy, buy refillable products or products in larger packaging as it's much more environmentally friendly. Glass is a far greener choice than plastic, so choose it wherever you can. If you want mini-versions for travelling light, simply refill from larger bottles rather than buying new.

520 USE TINTED GLASS

If you're storing essential oils for use around your home in the place of chemical cleaners and bathroom products, make sure you keep them in dark glass bottles as opposed to plastic. This protects the oils from sunlight and preserves their natural properties.

521 GET SALTY AT BATHTIME

Relax and unwind with bath salts instead of foaming bath oils and bubble baths, which can contain chemicals such as sodium laureth sulphate. They're a much greener choice.

522 SPEAK OUT

Take a stand by letting manufacturers who consistently over-package know that's the reason why you've stopped buying their products. There's nothing like purchasing power to force changes.

523 LIQUIDIZE YOUR ASSETS

Plastic soap dispensers are a great choice when it comes to hygiene but bad in terms of packaging. Make your own liquid soap by putting a bar of soap in boiling water and using the liquid to top up existing applicators.

524 STAMP OF APPROVAL

If your cream is USDA Organic Certified, you can be sure it's produced to organic standards. Other recognized brands are EcoCert, Soil Association and BioDynamic.

525 SOAP IT UP

For a green alternative to chemical-ridden cleaners that's kinder on your skin and the planet, mix 125 ml (4 fl oz) pure soap with 4 litres (7 pints) hot water and 50 ml (2 fl oz) lemon juice. For a stronger cleaner, double the amount of soap and lemon juice.

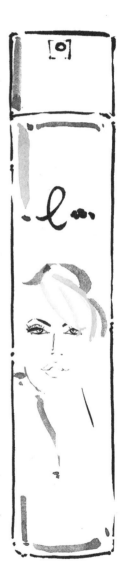

526 PUMP UP THE CAN

Wherever possible, choose pump action sprays for beauty products such as hair spray and leave-in conditioner rather than aerosol cans. Most products come in alternative packaging nowadays so there's really no excuse to buy an aerosol.

skin at work

527 KEEP IT SIMPLE

If you lead a busy life, the last thing you need is a complicated morning skincare routine. Keep it as simple and brief as you can, and leave the more time-consuming treatments and products for the evening.

528 USE AN SPF

You might think that because you don't spend much time outside during the day you can do without an SPF, but remember enough UV rays can pass through glass to cause skin damage. If you're travelling by car, bus or train, or sit near a window at work, add a layer of protection.

529 GET HUMID

A good way to increase the moisture in the air – which helps keep skin hydrated – at your desk is to invest in a mini-misting water feature for your desk, or club together with colleagues for a room humidifier. Or simply use a facial mist to help deliver a hydrating punch several times a day.

530 CLEAN YOUR KEYS

It's all too easy to forget about your keyboard when it comes to cleaning, but keyboards are a perfect breeding ground for germs, being touched by so many fingers. Clean at least once a week.

531 KEEP IT LIGHT

When it comes to make-up for the office, it's a good idea to keep things light. Thick layers of cosmetics are more prone to drying and flaking, while thinner layers can be refreshed with facial spritzes and moisturizers.

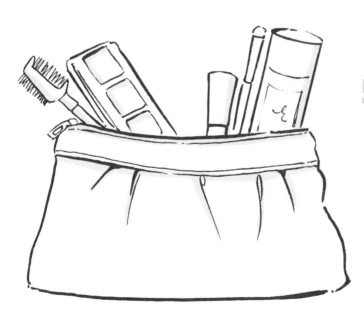

532 ALTER YOUR ENVIRONMENT

You might not be able to change how sunny it is, or how many pollutant toxins you're exposed to on the way to work, but you will have some control over the places were you spend most of your time: your bedroom, your home and your place of work. Aim to create a better environment for your skin by making those places work for rather than against it.

533 BLOT UP OIL

If you work in a large office with air conditioning, chances are the air will be dry enough to boost your skin's oil production. Keep blotting paper in your desk to prevent your face from shining.

534 USE A PROTECTIVE SERUM

To help prevent your skin from drying out at work, use a protective serum in the morning under your moisturizer and make-up. The best type of moisturizer to use for a day in the office is one designed to create a thin but breathable film on the top of the skin, which will hold in moisture but protect against damage and dryness.

535 CARRY A HAND CREAM

Your hands are just as prone to dryness in the office as your facial skin, but they're often neglected and – even worse – washed with harsh office soap. Take along your own hand cream to reapply during the day.

post-workout skin tips

536 GET ACTIVE

Exercising is one of the best things you can do for your skin – activity boosts the skin's blood flow, flooding it with oxygenated blood and helping it stay in top condition. Aim for three to four 30-minute workouts a week.

537 DRINK IT UP

The number one tip for keeping skin healthy while you work out is to make sure you stay hydrated by drinking lots of water. This will help keep your skin moisturized from the inside out.

538 WORK IT OFF

Sweating is a great way to help keep skin healthy, but it's important to make sure that you wash off the sweat afterwards as the salts it contains can help skin dry out. If you're not planning to shower, use fresh water to rinse skin afterwards, but cleanse for better results.

539 TAKE TWO TOWELS

Always wipe down equipment, before and after use. If possible, use two separate towels – one for wiping down machines and one for your face and body. Wash both after each visit.

540 GO LIGHT

Going bare faced for your workout is the best way to help your skin breathe. If you must wear a "face", use the lightest formula you can to allow your skin to sweat without drastic results! If you must wear make-up to the gym or while you exercise or dance, apply it an hour before you head off. That way you allow it time to set, which means it's less likely to start "sliding" as you heat up.

541 SEE A SERUM

If you're taking make-up off to work out but you have oily skin and you're concerned about it turning shiny, a good option is to use an oil-reducing serum. That way, you're putting a minimal amount of product onto your skin but you'll still look great.

542 THE EYES HAVE IT

A great way to keep your face made up while exercising but still give it a chance to "breathe" is to concentrate on eye make-up. Waterproof mascara and pencil draws attention to the eyes, allowing you to wear less, or no, make-up on the rest of your face.

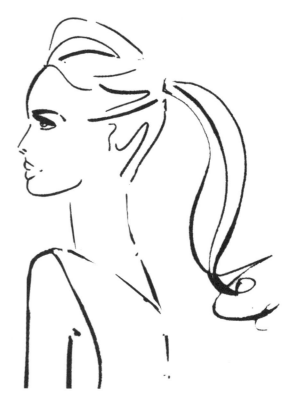

543 GO TINTED

It's not a good idea to use lipstick while working out as it can slip and slide; also, you're likely to smear it as you wipe your face. Instead choose lip gloss or a tinted chapstick to keep lips moisturized as well as coloured.

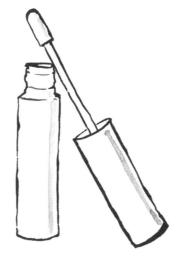

544 TIE IT BACK

Scrape hair back from your face when exercising to help reduce the amount you sweat and stop your face looking messy. If your hair is long enough for a ponytail or other up do, secure it well, or use a hairband or sweatband to keep your fringe tamed.

545 GO MILD

The key to your post-workout cleanse is to stay mild – it's important to wash off all those salts and minerals. Choose cleansers and body washes with a pH value of around 5.5 (similar to that of water itself) to minimize the drying effects and help skin stay hydrated.

546 SCREEN YOURSELF

If you're exercising outside, wearing a sunscreen is essential to help protect skin from damage and dryness, but sun creams are often heavy and greasy. Choose a specific waterproof and sweatproof face cream, or use gel or wipes for a lighter application.

547 TAKE IT OFF

Wearing a sports bra is essential to help reduce stretching of the skin due to bouncing boobs while working out, but the tightness can also trap sweat and bacteria, leading to skin problems. Change any tight clothing as soon as possible after exercise, preferably showering as well.

548 CAN'T STAND THE HEAT

Avoid a really hot shower or bath after a workout – choose warm or lukewarm water instead, as it will help the skin recover. If you can bear it, finish off with a splash of cool water to your face to help close up pores and stimulate blood flow.

travel tips

549 DAB-ON TOOTHPASTE

Toothpaste is a great on-the-spot treatment if you develop a blemish when you're away. It contains the antibacterial ingredient triclosan and it's also a drying agent, which can strip away excess oils.

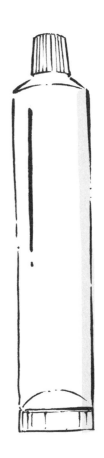

550 BE A WATER BABY

For every hour on board a flight you can lose 100 ml (3½ fl oz) of water from your skin. Stay hydrated by drinking at least 250 ml (8 fl oz) every hour and use a hydrating moisturizer while on board. Try to get some sleep, too, to allow skin to regenerate.

551 TRAVEL WELL

If you're out and about with work or children, take a mini on-the-go survival kit in your bag to help you look after your skin wherever you are. Travel sizes of cleansing wipes, hand cream, lip balm, spot treatment, cover up and illuminating face cream are all good choices.

552 SPRITZ YOURSELF

Humidity is usually less than 20 per cent inside an airplane, which is extremely dry. Freshen up your skin by splashing face with cold water or spritz regularly with water, mineral spritz or rosewater to tone the skin. Use an eye gel to help keep eyes hydrated too.

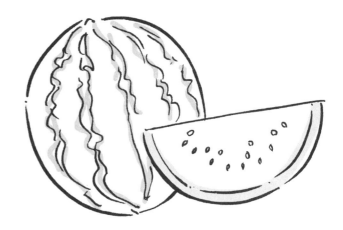

553 BEAT THE BLOAT

While travelling, your diet may contain salty or sugary foods, which can dehydrate your skin. Choose diuretic foods like watercress, watermelon, fennel and peppermint, which all reduce bloating and puffiness and help skin appear firmer and younger.

554 BOOK A TREATMENT

A number of airport spas and therapy centres have now opened up across the globe so you can indulge your skin prior to the dryness and dehydration of air travel. Book a hydrating facial before your flight to protect against damage.

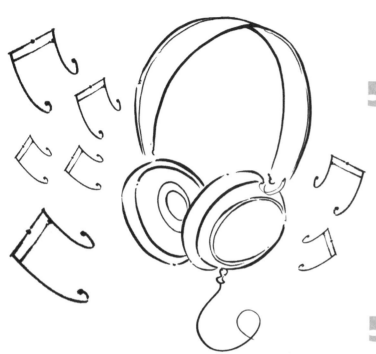

skincare for babies & children

556 CREATE WATER BABIES

Adult skin produces lots of oils which need cleansing at the end of the day, but until puberty children's skin produces remarkably little oil (which is why they rarely smell!), so there's no need to use lots of soap and other products in their bath. Apart from the face and hands, try using just water to cleanse every other day or use a soap-free emulsifying cleanser.

557 SUPPLEMENT THEIR DIET

Children's skin is particularly susceptible to damage, so make sure you feed your family a diet that is rich in antioxidants, and also consider giving your children a daily multivitamin supplement. Do check the container label, though, as many children's supplements contain artificial colours, flavourings and preservatives that can lessen the beneficial effects.

555 RELAX AND UNWIND

Try to relax your mind during your flight with lots of deep breathing and listening to music, but remember to move your body to prevent swelling and reduction in circulation. Aim to stand up and stretch every 45 minutes; walk around the plane or circle legs and ankles.

558 GET SOUR

If you are using cotton nappies (diapers) rather than disposables, rinse them in a vinegar and water solution after washing them to make the most of the anti-bacterial and anti-fungal properties of vinegar. Use the diluted mixture to dab onto nappy rash if you don't use cotton nappies.

559 THINK "BEENS"

When applying sunscreen to your children it's easy to miss areas like the backs of knees or the lower back. Coloured sunscreens are good for this, or apply liberally so you can see uncovered areas. Remember BEENS – Backs of knees, Ears, Eyes, Neck and Scalp.

560 GO OILY

For babies, avoid harsh products containing petrochemicals, even if labelled "mild" Instead, use a natural oil such as mild olive oil or almond oil (unless they have nut allergies) to massage and moisturize your baby's skin and leave it feeling soft and supple, not clogged.

561 SMOTHER WITH CALENDULA

Calendula cream (made from marigold flowers) is gentle and won't irritate your baby's delicate skin. It also helps the skin heal itself, so it's a great solution for nappy diaper) rash.

562 OPEN SESAME!

Sesame oil is a good moisturizer for the baby's nappy (diaper) area and it's light enough to be easily absorbed into the skin. Olive oil and almond oil are good alternatives and you can mix either of these with a little water to help thin them out further.

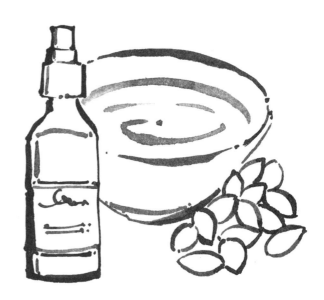

563 GET MILKY-SMOOTH

Breast milk is sterile as it leaves the body and it's a great moisturizer and skin freshener. Use breast milk (or regular milk, if you're bottle feeding) to massage into your child's bottom to reduce redness and pain.

564 BE PHTHALATE-FREE

Phthalates are substances found in many adult (and some baby) toiletries. There has been some suspicion that they can absorb into the skin and cause damage to very young children so many parents choose phthalate-free to be on the safe side.

565 SPOT THE DIFFERENCE

If your child develops a rash or spots on his skin don't assume it's an allergy. Consult a doctor to rule out harmless skin conditions such as water warts (*Molluscum contagiosum*), which causes hard, fluid-filled spots to appear for several months.

566 WASH HANDS THOROUGHLY

One of the healthiest habits you can pass on for your children's skin (and general) health is to teach them to wash their hands properly. They will avoid passing germs from hands to face and this sets up good habits for life.

567 ARM YOURSELF WITH ARNICA

Arnica is a great handbag essential for busy mums, especially during summer months when bumps and bruises are common. It's been shown to reduce the severity of bruising and helps calm inflamed skin.

teenage skin

568 B HEALTHY

Often teenage girls develop a skin condition known as "hormone-related acne", which is linked to the menstrual cycle. Both GLA (from evening primrose oil) and vitamin B6 are known to help prevent these problems. Encourage your child to take a supplement daily if you think this could be the cause.

569 OIL IT UP

Ironically, oily skin can benefit from more oil in the diet – so long as it's the right type. To redress the natural balance in your child's skin, encourage them to take linseed oil, borage (or starflower) oil or evening primrose oil supplements.

570 CHANGE YOUR ROUTINE

During puberty, both boys and girls start to produce more hormones, which can have an adverse effect on the skin. Boys are more prone to acne because androgens (the male hormones) increase the size of sebaceous glands and boost sebum production. Skin requires completely different attention during these times – more than likely the skincare regime will need to change completely.

571 SINK THE ZINC

Healthy skin requires a good dose of zinc to help control inflammation and skin repair. It is interesting that most acne sufferers are teenagers, whose zinc reserves may well be used up in growth spurts (something boys are more prone to than girls). Taking a supplement is the easiest way to keep levels topped up, ideally 45 mg a day.

572 AVOID THE FIZZ

It's just at the time when teenagers enter puberty that they start to have more control over their own diets. This can mean an increase in sugary snacks and fizzy drinks, which are high in phosphoric acid, which in turn can be detrimental to skin health. Encourage them to drink lots of water and snack on fruit instead.

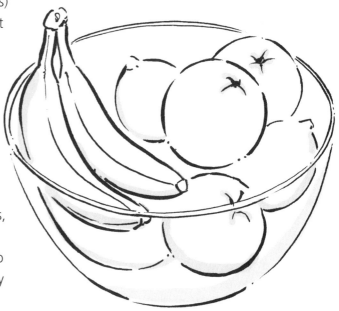

post-party remedies

573 DROP IT

Following a night out, eyes can often feel dry and sore, which makes the surrounding skin red and puffy. Use standard moisturizing eye drops to bring your whiteness back and help reduce trauma to the surrounding skin areas.

574 MASK THE PROBLEM

Applying a mask the morning after can help skin feel more alive by giving it a boost of vitamins and sloughing away dead skin cells. Choose a regenerating, moisturizing or brightening mask for these occasions, even if you would usually use a different type.

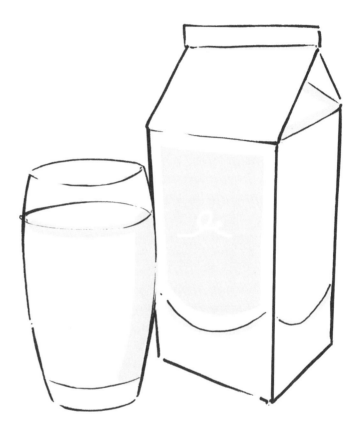

575 LOCK-IN MOISTURE

A good moisturizing cream is perfect for the morning after, but don't assume that the thicker the cream, the better it will be. Some of the most hydrating creams are lighter formulations with ingredients such as glycerin and vitamin E, rather than oil-based products.

576 GET MILKY WHITE

Soak cotton-wool balls or pads in ice-cold milk and apply to your eyes for a few minutes until they are warm. Repeat for at least five minutes and the milk will not only reduce puffiness but also help the whites of your eyes stay white.

577 EXFOLIATE, EXFOLIATE

Exfoliating skin the morning after can help remove any traces of the damaging stressors that might still be lurking on the skin's surface (especially if you were slightly lax about your cleansing before bed). Use a hot cloth rather than grainy face washes to avoid traumatizing the skin.

578 SAY EYE-EYE

Depuff tired eyes and reduce puffiness and under-eye circles by applying an eye gel, serum or cream, then lie back with a cold compress over your eyes for five to 10 minutes. The cooling feeling helps reduce fluid and blood flow to the area and also boosts the action of the cream.

579 BE A VIT CLEVER

If you've been burning the candle at both ends, chances are your skin is suffering a lack of antioxidant vitamins. Taking a glass of water with a soluble vitamin C tablet before bed can help because it balances the body as it rehydrates and reduces problems the morning after.

580 FAKE IT

People with paler skins can often look pallid and washed-out the morning after. Using a fake tan or bronzer gives a feel-good boost and evens out skin tone while you recover.

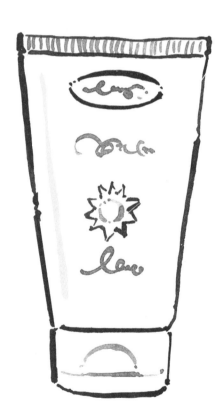

581 DO A DETOX

If your skin feels clogged and heavy after partying, choose products with detoxifying ingredients such as marigold, rosehip, St John's wort and jojoba, as well as tea tree and eucalyptus. Be sure to work from the inside out, too – take a daily vitamin supplement to ensure your skin gets sufficient nutrients.

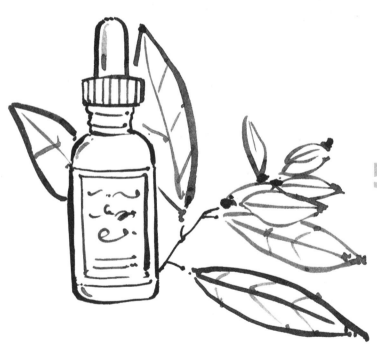

582 COOL IT

If you trust yourself to remember to remove your make-up before you go to bed, a great way to help your skin is to leave your products in the fridge before you leave for your night out. That way, when you come to use them they'll deliver a cooling effect as well as cleansing.

583 FEED YOUR SKIN

Choose creams and serums that soothe the skin and feed it with the nutrients that have been depleted by partying. Ingredients such as lavender, rose, aloe vera and camomile are all good boosters. Apply to cleansed skin before you go to sleep, and then again the morning after.

584 OIL AWAY PROBLEMS

If your skin tends to look pallid the morning after – perhaps more grey than pink – use a facial oil the night before to help regenerate and bring back your usual rosy complexion. Choose ingredients that deliver a moisture punch and contain soothing, anti-inflammatory properties.

585 PARTY TIME

If the party season is upon you, it's likely you'll be going out more than once or twice a week and so your skin will need even more attention. Plan at least one 24-hour period at home without make-up, where you can really attend to your skin. A face mask, foot cream, no salt, sugar or alcohol plus a good night's sleep helps keep skin healthy through the hammering.

586 SIP A PIP

Lemon juice contains high levels of vitamin C, but almost certainly the last thing you want to do the morning after is to start eating a lemon. Steal a tip from the celebrities and make yourself a morning beauty booster. Stir the juice of half a lemon into warm water to boost vitamin levels; it also acts as a detoxifier and helps clear membranes.

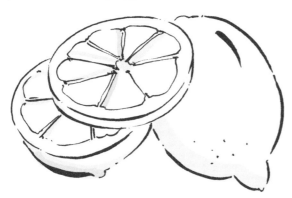

587 DRINK IT UP

Our skin is comprised mainly of water, and it's the first bit of the body to dehydrate after a big night out. Drinking enough water the night before (alternate water with other drinks) is the best way to avoid it. In the morning try alternating a glass of plain filtered water with an electrolyte-balanced energy drink to avoid diluting the body's natural salts and minerals.

588 KEEP CLEAN

While you sleep, the skin is most receptive to soaking up products from the surface of the skin, and if the surface of your skin is covered in stale cigarette smoke, make-up, sweat and environmental toxins, that's what you'll be feeding your skin. Always cleanse before you go to sleep – even a quick rub with a cleansing wipe will work. Leave some beside your bed before you go out to remind you.

pregnancy & post-pregnancy

588 MAKE A CHANGE

Hormones change completely during pregnancy and again while breastfeeding. If your skin type changes, don't hang onto old habits but adapt to your new skin and develop a new routine with different products.

589 E-RASE STRETCH MARKS

The best creams for preventing stretch marks are those containing collagen and elastin. If stretch marks have already appeared, however, smother with vitamin E cream and rub in gently twice a day to help prevent scarring and encourage regeneration.

591 ANTI-STRETCH STRIVECTIN

StriVectin is a formulation in face and body creams that includes skin-firming agents, elasticizers and skin hydrators. It has been shown to lead to visible stretch mark and wrinkle reduction.

592 TEND YOUR EXTREMITIES

Your extremities – the hands, feet, lower legs and lower arms – are often neglected by the circulation system during pregnancy because the body is concentrating on the growing foetus. Be sure to give them extra care – gentle exercise and massage can help boost circulation and keep the skin healthy and supple.

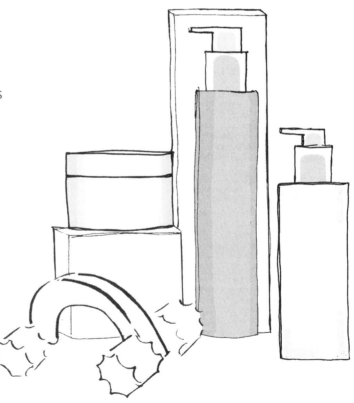

593 MAKE MINE A MARIGOLD

Pregnant skin is more prone to bruising than at any other time because of the increased blood flow in the body. Use arnica cream to help reduce bruising or make up your own bruise-busting infusion with a handful of marigold flowers steeped in 300 ml (½ pint) of boiled water. Leave to steep for 15 minutes, then wipe onto the affected area.

594 FEED YOUR SKIN

During pregnancy the body's basal metabolic rate increases and as skin is an organ, the turnover of skin cells increases too. Therefore, it's even more important to exfoliate regularly and to moisturize to keep skin supple, especially in those areas that will expand considerably, such as the abdomen, breasts and hips.

595 INSTANT COOL-DOWN

If your ankles, feet and legs suffer from the heat in summer, invest in a pair of aloe vera-infused tights. Their heat-reducing action makes them a cooler choice than bare legs, helping skin stay cooler too.

596 BE PATIENT WITH PIGMENT

Because the body's hormones change so dramatically during pregnancy, many women find their skin pigment changes too (a condition called chloasma). Don't be too hasty in seeking treatment, though – just keep the area well moisturized and healthy, and it should return to normal a few months after the birth.

597 RUB YOUR BUMP

During pregnancy the skin has a lot of stretching to do but it's often lacking in vitamins because the body uses so many to grow the baby. Massaging your belly daily with oil or cream delivers a vitamin boost to the skin and keeps it supple and hydrated, as well as reducing itching and discomfort.

598 DON'T BE AN A-STUDENT

Increased hormone levels mean pregnant women are more prone to spots, especially during the first few months. Beware of products containing vitamin A, such as Retin-A, which can cause problems for the developing foetus. Seek medical advice first.

599 BANISH BERGAMOT

Bergamot essential oil is often prescribed to ease relaxation of muscles during pregnancy but it can lead to the skin developing areas of uneven pigmentation, especially during pregnancy or when the sun is shining. Opt for other citrus-based oils instead.

menopause

600 BE AN ICE BABE

Try products based on glacial minerals to calm skin and soothe inflammation. Willow bark is also a great choice as it contains natural salicylic acid to soothe irritation and prevent breakouts and congestion.

601 PHYT AGEING

Phytoestrogens, which are hormone-like substances produced by plants, are a great way to help reduce the effects of the menopause. Soy is particularly rich in genistein and daidzein, two substances that mimic the effects of oestrogen in the body.

602 STEP BACK IN TIME

Because one of the major symptoms of menopause is a reduction is oestrogen, the body becomes more susceptible to the oily skin effects of the male hormones, which means acne-like blemishes can develop during menopause exactly as in puberty. Think back to your youth – the targeted spot treatments that worked for you then could be just as effective now.

603 PEEL IT

Having a facial peel is another good choice during menopause as the skin is often dryer and subject to build-up of dry skin, even if you exfoliate regularly. Regular peels can encourage regeneration and avoid the skin dryness many women suffer.

604 GET HANDY

Hands-on therapies such as massage are a great choice for menopause because they help reduce aches and pains. In addition, they boost circulation and lymphatic drainage, giving skin an oxygen boost and reducing inflammation.

605 DO SOME YOGA

Practising yoga and other deep breathing techniques can help to boost circulation and balance hormone levels in the body, so increasing oxygenation and reducing breakouts. Three times a week is ideal.

606 KEEP IT WARM

A soothing evening bath is a great way to unwind and give your skin a treat, but during the menopause you might have to tone down the heat. Hot water can have a drying effect on the skin, too, so go for warm instead.

607 JOIN THE JUNIPER

If you suffer aching joints and skin problems during menopause, try adding some juniper to your bath to help draw out toxins from the skin. Afterwards, use a light hydrating moisturizer if you have normal skin, or an oil if skin is dry and thirsty.

608 GET ESSENTIAL

During menopause, swap your usual aromatherapy choices for oils with specific menopausal benefits – choose clary sage, geranium, lavender, neroli, peppermint, lemon, jasmine and camomile.

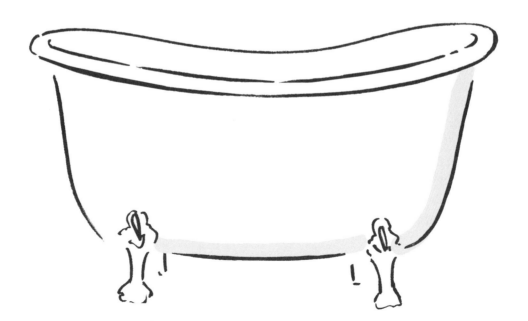

608 CHANGE YOUR CREAM

Oestrogen is also responsible for stimulating the production of hyaluronic acid, which keeps skin hydrated and smooth. After the menopause skin is likely to be dryer and less able to hold onto moisture, as well as being thinner as regeneration also slows down. Dramatic changes in skincare regimes are required, with the use of heavier, more hydrating creams.

610 CHANGE CATEGORY

After the menopause, most women's skin needs move from "anti-ageing" to "ageing" when it comes to products. You might still feel young, but your skin needs different things now the body's oestrogen levels are lower, so switch products straight away.

611 EYES RIGHT

As skin starts to get thinner after the menopause, veins under the skin (especially around the eyes) become more visible. Using an eye cream is essential to help keep skin hydrated, as well as under-eye concealer or light diffuser.

men only

612 LUBE YOUR FACE

If you have sensitive skin but need to shave daily, watch out for razor bumps. These can look like acne but are in fact caused when the newly-cut sharp ends of the hair grow down or along into the skin and cause a swelling. Use a lubricating shaving gel and a sharp razor.

613 SHAVE DOWN

Whatever area of the body you are shaving, always shave downward in the direction of hair growth rather than against the hair, which can cause bumps and swelling. After shaving, splash with cold water or use an oil-free moisturizer.

614 ACNE-PROTECTOR

If you suffer from acne, shaving can be difficult. Look for a lubricating but non-clogging shaving gel or a prescription shaving foam containing benzoyl peroxide that's designed specifically for men suffering from acne.

615 SMOOTH OPERATOR

If you're going to have a facial treatment at a salon, don't shave immediately beforehand because this can leave the skin tender and less receptive to products. If your treatment is in the morning, try shaving the night before, or that morning if it's an afternoon appointment.

616 STAY SHARP

Shaving can be good for acne as it acts as a natural exfoliant and opens up pores to drain away excess oil, but if you traumatize the skin by using a blunt or dirty razor, it can make matters worse. Always choose a fresh, sharp razor and clean it carefully after use.

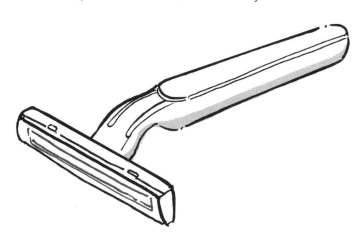

617 LEAVE THE BAR EARLY

Many men make the mistake of assuming that using an ordinary body soap bar in the shower is OK for their face too, but the soap can actually strip away natural oils from the sensitive skin of your face. Use a facial cleanser instead.

618 GET MOISTURIZED

Don't make the mistake of thinking that as men's skin is thicker, it doesn't need moisturizing. Men's facial skin is often very dehydrated, especially with all that shaving. If your skin ever feels tight after washing, this means there's not enough water in it. Moisturize after shaving in the morning and last thing at night.

619 COLD SPLASH

At the end of your shave rinse a washcloth in cold water and press to the shaved area to help reduce blood flow and close pores. This minimizes the likelihood of you developing shaving rash and infections, and reduces any redness and swelling too. Splashing your face with cold water also works.

620 SCRUB IT OFF

Scrub your face with an exfoliant or face cloth a couple of times a week to help prevent dry, flaky skin from clogging the skin's surface and reduce the chance of ingrown hairs after shaving. But don't take the word "scrub" too literally: your touch should be firm but not enough to pull or scratch your skin. Concentrate on the areas you don't shave – they are likely to have more dry skin build-up.

621 BE PATIENT

If possible, wait about 30 minutes after getting up in the morning before shaving because this allows the facial muscles to tighten and means the hair is more likely to stand up from the skin for a smoother finish. Before you begin, gently rub the areas you plan to shave.

622 PRESS THE FLESH

To soften skin and hairs to help you achieve a closer, smoother shave, soak a warm facecloth in warm water. Press onto the skin for several minutes first.

623 QUALITY, NOT QUANTITY

When it comes to shaving foam, less is more. Use less of the actual product and lather it up with vigorous rubbing rather than using lots of product, which the razor might struggle to get through. Rinse often during the shave to ensure the foam doesn't clog up the razor.

624 WORK OUT TO IN

The best way to shave is jawline and cheeks first, then move in towards the lips, neck and chin, where the hair is thickest. Shaving can take off the top layers of skin, so avoid going over the same area more than once or twice to reduce redness.

625 GET YOUR OWN

The best thing to do if you want to moisturize or cleanse your face with something other than shower gel or soap is to invest in a product designed especially for men. These are more likely to contain ingredients particular to male skincare needs. Leave your partner's products alone!

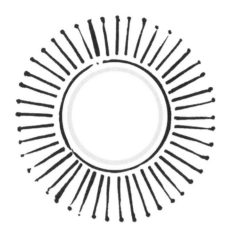

tattoos & piercings

628 TRY BEFORE YOU BUY

Considering a tattoo? Don't forget it's a decision for life so think carefully; do your research on the type of tattoo and where to have it done. Getting a temporary tattoo of the design you want and living with it for a few weeks or months is a great way to help you decide if permanent ink will really suit your lifestyle.

626 BLOCK OUT THE SUN

Men are twice as likely to get skin cancer than women, probably because they are less likely to wear sunscreen or seek shade. Choosing a morning moisturizer with added SPF is a great way to keep your skin protected for everyday activities, but you'll need more than that if you're sunbathing.

629 GET A TEST

Always ask for a patch test before you have a tattoo, especially if you're having coloured ink that's green, blue or yellow, which can cause allergic skin reactions.

627 KEEP IT CLEAN

Razors should always be kept clean and free of hair and products. Store upright with the blades facing upwards, not blade down as this can cause bluntness and damage the skin. If you have changeable blades, aim to do this every week.

630 THINK MEDICAL

If you have medical issues that might involve having a lot of MRI scans, speak to your doctor before having a tattoo. Some of the inks used in permanent make-up and tattoos can interfere with the scanner.

631 SCAR BABY

If your skin is prone to scarring in keloid lumps rather than flat, then think twice about having a tattoo, which relies on the body's scarring system to remain permanent. Discuss the right choice for your skin with a reputable tattoo clinic.

632 FUTURE PLANS

When choosing a tattoo, always think about whether or not you want it to be covered by clothes, possible changes in career that might prove problematic in the future, and changes in body shape (for instance, pregnancy stretches the skin of your abdomen).

633 GO REPUTABLE

Always choose a reputable, licensed tattoo studio employing properly trained staff. Check with your local health department or council for registered places to get inked. And don't be afraid to ask questions before you book – any reputable studio will be pleased to show you how careful they are about hygiene.

634 GET THEM TO GLOVE UP

Don't be afraid to ask your tattoo artist or piercer to wash their hands and wear gloves before working on your tattoo. If you feel at all uneasy, remember you're paying for their service – you can always change your mind and leave if you get the feeling it's not clean enough.

635 CHECK THE SEAL

Before any procedure begins, make sure you see your tattoo artist or piercer remove the needles and tubes from sealed packages. Any pigments, trays, containers and washes should also be unused. Don't be afraid to ask them to change equipment if you're at all unsure.

636 DON'T DIY

Some home-use creams claim to help remove tattoos by breaking down the pigment in the tattoo and allowing it to fade into the skin, but there's not a lot of evidence they do anything more than fade the ink. They can cause skin reactions too, so it's always best to see a professional.

637 FIND THE AUTOCLAVE

If you're having a tattoo or piercing and the person performing the procedure is using non-disposable equipment, make sure they use a heat sterilization machine (an autoclave) to thoroughly sterilize equipment to remove harmful germs and bacteria. Equipment that cannot be sterilized should be disinfected after each use.

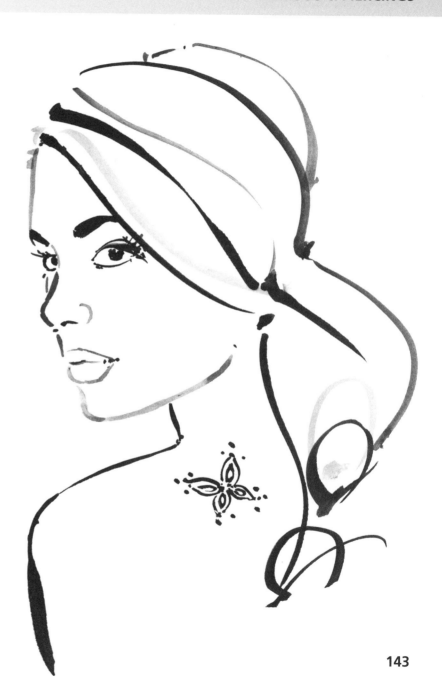

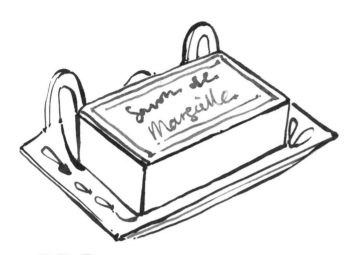

640 KEEP IT MOIST

Once you are sure the skin is not broken, apply a mild, fragrance-free moisturizer to the tattooed area several times a day to keep skin supple and encourage it to heal. Or go for mild, natural moisturizers such as olive or almond oil.

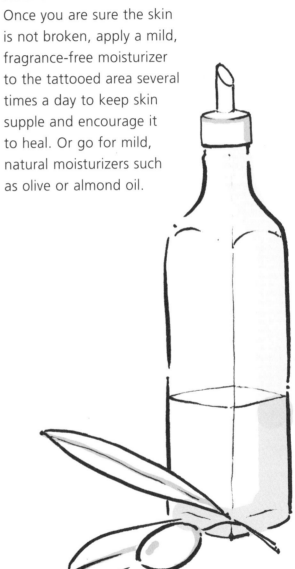

638 BE GENTLE

Use plain soap or body wash and warm water to cleanse a newly applied tattoo but avoid standing under the shower or rubbing with a towel. In short the gentler you are with your tattoo, the better it will heal. Allow two weeks for total healing.

639 GO ANTIBIOTIC

If you've had a tattoo or piercing, remove the bandage after about 24 hours and apply an antibiotic ointment to protect against infection. Don't fiddle with the tattoo and remember, rough clothing could cause irritation and infection.

144

641 NO SWIMMING

Keep your new tattoo or piercing out of the sun and away from harsh chemicals such as those in swimming pool water. Also, steer clear of pools, hot tubs, rivers, lakes and the sea to avoid infection while you have broken skin.

642 LASER IT OFF

Some tattoos are easier to remove by laser surgery than others – those with fewer colours mixed together are simplest as the laser targets specific colour wavelengths (red and black are easiest to remove). Most tattoos require six to eight treatments, three to four weeks apart, for 80 to 90 per cent clearance. Treated areas may blister, burn and even bleed, with skin crusting for several days and there could be some scarring.

643 GO HYPO

If your skin is at all sensitive, make sure your piercer uses hypoallergenic jewellery. Nickel can cause allergic reactions in some people, so look for surgical-grade steel, titanium, niobium or 14- or 18-carat gold.

644 WASH YOUR MOUTH OUT

If you've had a piercing in your mouth, lip, cheek or tongue, use an antibacterial, alcohol-free mouthwash to keep it clean (or for a milder alternative, rinse with packaged sterile saline). Rinse for at least 30 seconds after each meal and before you go to bed.

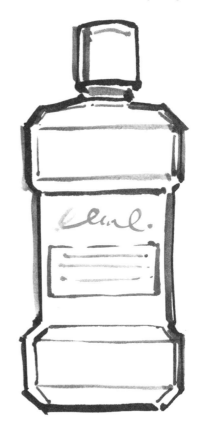

anti-ageing habits

645 SAFEGUARD SENIOR SKIN

The skin on your face is the thinnest on the body and the older it is, the thinner and drier it will be. It needs extra protection and moisture, especially during the harsh winter months, so moisturize frequently and avoid harsh toners.

646 DON'T MAKE THE FACE

Making faces and adopting signature facial expressions creates folds and wrinkles between the brows and eyes. Simply being aware of your facial expressions, particularly in the sun, will prevent them from appearing in the first place.

647 THINK MORE OR LESS

As you get older, your skin changes and is less able to take heavy make-up. Your rule of thumb should be to use more skin-helping products like night creams and anti-ageing serums and lighter make-up.

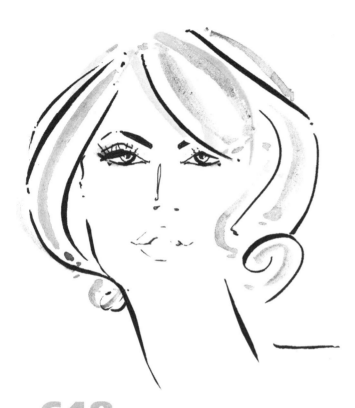

648 APPLY LESS COLOUR

As skin ages, it is also likely to change in colour and in most people this means less definition between the different areas such as lips, eyes, cheeks and hair. Often older skin looks better with more natural shades to reflect this. If you're a fan of colour, try to temper the shades a bit to avoid an unnatural look.

649 KNOW YOUR NASTIES

If you're worried about chemicals and toxins in products, the main ones to steer clear of on ingredients lists are: propylene glycol (used in antifreeze), isopropyl alcohol, methylisothiazolinone, sodium lauryl sulphate (used in engine degreaser), formaldehyde, stearalkonium chloride, DEA (diethanolamine) and TEA (triethanolamine).

650 FIGHT FREE RADICALS

Free radicals, small unstable oxygen molecules, attach to other cells of the body and break them down. Collagen is particularly susceptible to free radicals, which makes them stiff and less mobile. Eating foods rich in antioxidants and using skin products containing antioxidants can help reduce free radicals.

651 SMOOTH AWAY FINE LINES

To prevent ageing and ensure the delicate skin around your eyes stays taut, apply an eye cream above and below the eye area, morning and night, after the age of 25.

652 SPOT YOUR SKIN TYPE

Chronologically aged skin is a result of natural internal factors and manifests itself as thinner and less elastic skin that is otherwise smooth and unblemished. Photo-aged skin is marked by wrinkles, age spots, uneven pigmentation and a more leathery appearance, however.

653 START EARLY

Many of us think of anti-ageing products as being targeted toward much older, post-menopausal women but anti-ageing therapies and products are mostly preventative rather than curative. This means they're actually designed for women between the ages of 30 and 60.

654 GET YOUR BEAUTY SLEEP

Sleep is one of the best ways to reduce the signs of ageing as it allows the skin to replenish itself overnight. If you can't sleep, make sure your room isn't too hot – the deepest sleep occurs if your atmospheric temperature is 18–24°C (64–75°F).

655 KEEP HYDRATED

With age, cells stop regenerating at the rate they once did and in the same efficient way. As a result the skin's texture and water-retaining ability is diminished. The recommended daily intake of water is 2 litres (3½ pints) a day for women and 3 litres (5 pints) for men.

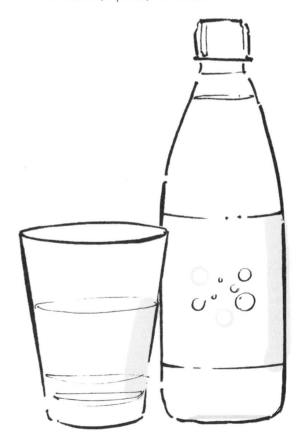

656 FAT LOSS MAKES YOU LOOK OLDER

As you age the underlying supportive fat tissues decrease, facial muscles become slacker and bone deteriorates, so the structure on which the skin sits becomes weaker. Losing too much weight as you age can make you look older.

657 ARREST PREMATURE AGEING

Rescue ageing skin by being scrupulous about using a sunscreen daily, keep out of the sun as much as possible and rescue early fine lines with intensive serums and brightening AHAs. You must use an SPF 15 in combination with acids such as AHA and BHA.

658 WEAR A MICRO MINERAL

Micronized titanium and zinc oxide mineral make-up provides sun protection and minimizes itching and burning. Due to the fact that these powders are composed entirely of micronized rock, they cannot grow bacteria, which makes them safe for use on sensitive, ageing and healing skin.

658 GIVE YOURSELF A HAND

Hands are one of the great giveaways of age. Look after your skin by wearing protective gloves when doing chores such as gardening or washing up and always use a hand cream containing UV filters during the day.

anti-ageing nutrition

660 EAT YOUR OLIVES

Olives – and olive oil – contain high levels of the phytonutrient squalene, which is thought to give skin a quick hydration boost because it's quickly absorbed into all skin layers.

661 GET A B-GRADE

To reduce wrinkles and dehydration, boost collagen production and increase the number of new cells your skin produces, optimize the B vitamins in your diet. Milk, eggs and fish are all good sources.

662 AN APPLE A DAY

Apples contain a veritable feast of antioxidants, which can help prevent the signs of ageing skin, such as dehydration and discoloration. Eating an apple a day is a great idea but make sure you don't discard the peel, which is where the benefits are mostly concentrated.

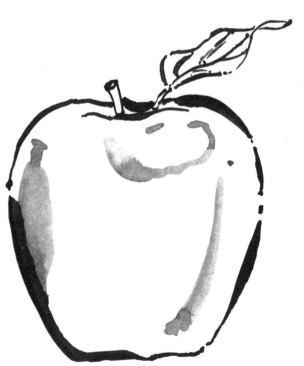

663 PICK UP PYCNOGENOL

Pycnogenol is an antioxidant found in pine bark that contains vitamins A, C and E, as well as its own age-busters. It is claimed to reverse and prevent wrinkles, so look out for it on ingredient lists for an anti-ageing boost.

664 REACH FOR RIBOSE

As your body ages, organs have less energy. Ribose is a naturally occurring "energy-booster" product which maximizes the efficiency of your skin cells, helping them to maximize the energy available to them for regrowth and regeneration, and thereby reducing the signs of ageing.

665 E'S ARE GOOD

Vitamin E, which is often found in products as Tocopherol, is one of the simplest and most potent anti-ageing ingredients around. It's particularly important during summer time and for people who spend lots of time outdoors, as vitamin E is reduced with prolonged sun exposure. Use vitamin E cream to limit wrinkles due to sun damage.

anti-ageing products

666 GET IN THE RETIN

Retin-A, a derivative compound from vitamin A, has been used to treat acne since it was first discovered in the 1960s. It has the ability to encourage the skin to regenerate, causing lower layers to grow faster. In high doses it can cause flaking, itching and dryness, though, so choose a low-potency cream to help even out skin tone, pigment, texture and growth.

667 PICK A PEPTIDE

Peptides are short-chain amino acids that are small enough to penetrate the top layers of skin. They can be chemically altered so they perform specific tasks in the skin, such as encouraging healing or boosting collagen production. Peptides are expensive but they're excellent for slowing the ageing process.

668 GO ALPHA

Alpha-lipoic acid, also known as lipoic acid, is soluble in both water and oil so it can penetrate the entire skin cell to deliver its antioxidant effect. It can also stimulate the production of collagen.

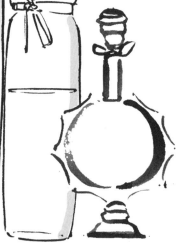

668 GO GLYCOLIC

Glycolic acid and other fruit acids are a great choice for anti-ageing products because they improve the smoothness and texture of skin by sloughing away the top layers and boosting regeneration. Over-the-counter creams containing these are often very low potency, however; salon-grade products are often more effective.

670 SHOW YOUR CERAMIDES

Ceramides are lipids (cellular fats) located in between skin cells to hold them together, keep pathogens (germs that cause disease) out and moisture in. Products containing ceramides aim to help repair this barrier to protect skin and prevent dehydration.

671 ACT YOUR AGE

Glycation is a process that occurs in the body whereby sugars and fats join to proteins and prevent the skin's natural regeneration from occurring as effectively as previously. Some products are now designed to soak up the Advanced Glycation End Products (Anti-AGE) to help protect collagen.

672 VIE FOR VITAMINS

Antioxidant vitamins C and E, and Co-enzyme Q10 can prevent sun damage, reverse problematic skin and boost the regeneration process. Instead of stripping away layers of skin like other anti-ageing ingredients, vitamins build it up. Although it might be tempting to go for a rich, oily cream, vitamins are often better delivered to the skin in a lighter formula.

673 KNOW THE SCORE

If your skin is scarred and/or ageing, choose products containing L-ascorbic acid, which is a highly stable form of vitamin C that boosts the synthesis of collagen to reduce the signs of damage and ageing.

674 BET A DIME

Dimethylaminoethanol is a synthetic compound naturally produced in the brain and also found in fish oil. It can increase muscle tone and therefore decreases the appearance of sagging, especially in combination with exfoliants such as hyaluronic acid.

675 COP SOME COPPER

Studies have shown that copper peptide in products can stimulate the production of structural fibres (including collagen and elastin). It can also enhance the body's ability to heal scars and wounds.

676 TEA TIME

Green tea extract is a powerful photo-protective agent, which means it can help protect skin against sun damage. Look for concentrations of 5 per cent for the best effects in skin products, or aim to drink two cups a day.

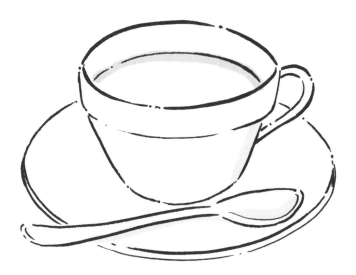

677 GO MOROCCAN

One of the best-kept skincare secrets to emerge in recent years is argan oil, which is produced from the kernels of the nuts of the argan tree, endemic to Morocco. Uniquely adapted to the dry, arid environment, the oil produced from argan nuts is thought to help skin heal and restore itself, reducing fine lines and wrinkles. It's also used in hair treatments.

678 SHIELD YOURSELF

Astaxanthin is a pigment that shields the skin and eyes of wild salmon from UV damage. It is now used in a range of anti-ageing products and serums to help reduce damage and pigmentation and also prevents fine lines and wrinkles due to its powerful antioxidant effects.

679 BE AN ANTI-AGEING PRO

Propolis is a resinous substance produced by some trees to protect them against environmental damage and is known for its anti-inflammatory and anti-ageing properties. The extract is included in skin creams.

680 GET SOME GROWTH

Some of the more hi-tech skincare products may contain proteins to stimulate cell growth and repair. These growth factor blends are listed on labels of products as PSP (processed skin cell proteins), TNS or TGF, and can help the skin appear visibly smoother and tighter by stimulating its self-healing capacities.

681 GO KOJIC FOR AGE SPOTS

Treat skin discoloration, such as freckles and age spots, with kojic acid. Discovered in Japan in 1989, kojic acid is derived from fungi. Gentle on the skin, it rebalances upper skin layers to inhibit uneven pigment formation. Results can be seen after four to six weeks.

682 TURN TO TURMERIC

The Indian spice turmeric, derived from the plant *Curcuma longa*, has antioxidant, exfoliating and anti-inflammatory properties which can help reverse the signs of ageing, including lines, wrinkles and saggy skin. It is also thought to brighten dark patches of pigment by eliminating melanocytes.

683 BE CERTAIN ABOUT SIRTUINS

Sirtuins are cellular proteins that are thought to have a central role in regulating the ageing process. They aim to promote cell repair and production of antioxidants by "switching on" the anti-ageing mechanisms.

684 DAY TO DAY

Day creams for anti-ageing should always contain a sunscreen that concentrates on blocking out the damaging, ageing UVA rays known to cause wrinkles and dryness in all skin types, but especially as it matures. Always use a day cream with SPF 15, whatever the weather.

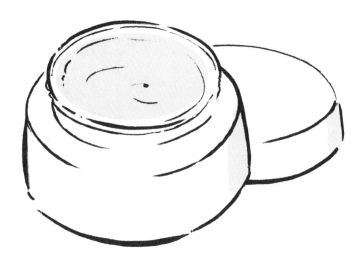

685 BRIGHTEN WITH DIOIC

A relatively new scientific compound known as dioic acid, also listed on ingredients labels as octadecenoic acid, has been shown to brighten hyperpigmentation or sun-damaged skin. The jury's still out on what concentration is best, but around 2 per cent is probably about right.

686 BE A CARNO-VORE

Carnosine is an amino acid that is needed to make muscle tissue in the body, but it's also a powerful antioxidant and anti-inflammatory agent. In addition, it protects and restores collagen, to slow down the ageing process, so it's a great choice for anti-ageing products.

687 GET SOME GROWTH

A new ingredient for anti-ageing and age-reversal creams is EGF (Epidermal Growth Factor), which is a synthesized compound made up of amino acids designed to stimulate collagen growth and cell renewal, leading to fewer wrinkles and fine lines and an increase in healing.

688 PICK THE STEM

The use of stem cell technology is still extremely controversial, especially in skincare products, but some products now include plant based stem cell products, which are believed to help heal skin and protect against ageing.

689 BE FRANK ABOUT AGEING

Frankincense is thought to have some anti-ageing properties by plumping up the skin and forming a protective barrier against further damage and stress. You'll find it in specialist creams and salon treatments.

690 GRAB A GLYCAN

Glycans are substances that are naturally present in the skin's cells, which are responsible for carrying the "youth" regeneration message to skin cells. As skin ages, they diminish and the cells regenerate less effectively. (You'll find them in serums such as YSL Forever Youth Liberator.)

681 SAVE THE PEEL

Apples are renowned for their antioxidant properties but it's the peel that contains the highest level of vitamins and minerals. The antioxidant compound phloretin is derived from apple skin and as well as an antioxidant, it works to reduce the signs of ageing and protects collagen.

682 RUMBA WITH KOMBUCHA

Kombucha tea is a highly nutritious black tea that delivers powerful antioxidant effects. It's an ingredient found in some anti-ageing skincare products to protect against dehydration and ageing, or can be used alone as a facial wash.

683 CRACK AN EGG

You will often see egg oil on the ingredients list for anti-ageing products. It's an occlusive agent, which means it helps the lubrication and texture of the cream and reduces degradation, which could lead to free radicals being released.

684 BAG A MULBERRY

Mulberry extract is thought to have pigment-levelling properties, helping the skin to re-distribute pigment to avoid patchy colouration. Look for it in combination with vitamin A for an even stronger effect.

anti-ageing therapies

685 GO FOR GABA

GABA is a surface-applied ingredient used pharmaceutically to freeze muscles, mimicking the effects of Botox without an invasive injection.

686 GET A HYDROXY PROXY

Alpha hydroxy acids and Beta hydroxy acids are chemical peels which help dissolve or degenerate the glue that holds the dead cells together on the skin, resulting in exfoliation of the top layers. Younger, newer skin cells are exposed and dryness and wrinkles reduced.

687 CHOOSE CACI

Caci facials tighten and tone skin by lifting muscles using the naturally occurring bio-electric current of the body to activate sagging muscles and skin tissue. Although expensive, the benefits can be seen after several treatments. It isn't just used for tightening facial lines – it can also be used to create a non-surgical bust lift by targeting sagging skin on the chest and lifting the bust.

688 BOOST YOUR OXYGEN

A great salon choice is a facial designed to boost the oxygen levels in your skin, known as oxygen therapy. Unavailable on the high street, these products combat damage caused by pollution and excessive lifestyles to leave skin feeling rejuvenated.

689 FILL IN LINES

The most popular filler is restylane, which is used to fill individual wrinkles or to plump up areas of the face; it's injected into the tissues. Purlane is a stronger form of filler, often used when people have lost a lot of weight to counteract the "hollow-cheeked" look.

700 BOX THE BOTOX

There are varying degrees of Botox because the more of the toxin injected into your body, the stronger the effects. Start off by asking your therapist for a very mild dose, which won't paralyse too many muscles; build up with subsequent treatments if you choose.

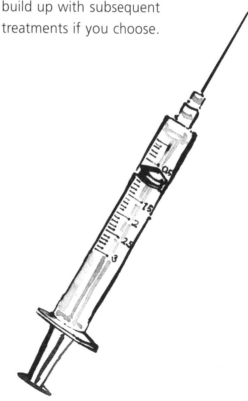

701 UNDERSTAND FRACTIONS

Fractional resurfacing is a laser treatment that works by targeting specific areas of skin rather than the whole skin surface. It's therefore a great choice for treating problem skin areas.

702 GET HEATED

Heat therapies, such as radiofrequency skin tightening, are designed to improve multiple areas of skin on the face, such as the forehead, jawline and neck. The heat is intense so it's preceded by a cooling gel and pain medication; it could be uncomfortable for a while afterwards.

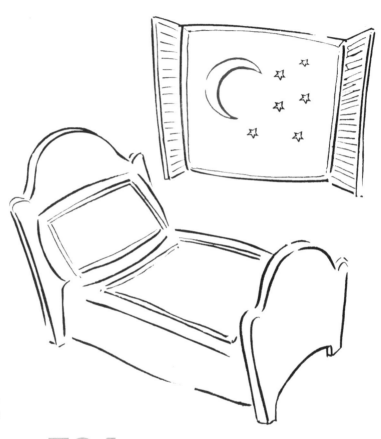

wrinkles & lines

703 WALK WRINKLES AWAY

Walking delivers oxygen to the complexion, gets the blood flowing and reduces tension-related wrinkles because it releases feel-good chemicals in the body. These in turn reduce stress and boost relaxation.

704 SILK SIREN

For the smoothest facial skin, copy the Egyptian queens and insist on a silk or satin pillow! It will smooth out facial wrinkles while you sleep and ensure you wake up looking your best.

705 KNOW YOUR WRINKLES

There are four different types of wrinkles – fine, deep, static and dynamic. Fine wrinkles, around the eyes, occur gradually due to the breakdown of collagen and elastin. Deeper ones, such as forehead lines, start in the muscles below the surface. Dynamic lines are those seen only when your face moves, while static wrinkles are seen all the time.

706 DON'T CONFUSE WRINKLES WITH DRYNESS

Dry skin can look more wrinkled, but actual wrinkles are not due to dry skin. These occur after damage to the skin's under-layers caused by ageing, sun exposure and smoking, as well as other pollutants.

707 BE COOL IN SHADES

Sunglasses stop lines caused by squinting against sun or harsh light from developing around your eyes. Watch out for changes in light intensity between inside and outside, and wear shades in winter, when the sun is lower, and also for driving.

708 REPAIR YOUR SKIN

Vitamin A can help diminish wrinkle depth, as its light inflammatory action "puffs up" the skin, so wrinkles appear less deep. You'll find it in anti-wrinkle creams. Alternatively, add it to your diet by eating lots of fruit and vegetables.

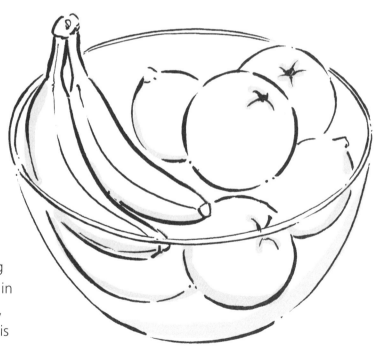

709 WHITE AND GREEN TEA

Green and white tea can help delay collagen ageing and weakening, which has been shown to be a premier cause of wrinkles. Many face creams use green and white tea, not only for their antioxidant properties but also because white tea is shown to limit DNA damage in sun-exposed skin. White tea also promotes new cell growth and strengthens the skin.

710 KEEP YOUR BROWLINE FREE

Squinting is a common cause of wrinkles, as muscles adapt to regular face positions. Wear glasses or contacts to avoid squinting and smooth out your forehead instead of frowning when you're upset or annoyed.

711 WITCH-HAZEL FACE FIRMER

Witch hazel temporarily tightens the skin to give facial tissues a lift. Instead of using it neat, which can stress delicate skin, mix 1 teaspoon with 100 g (3½ oz) of moisturizer and after two weeks you should see results.

712 WATERPROOF YOUR SKIN

Older skin needs a protective barrier to guard against cold weather and moisture loss. Look for a humectant cream that provides environmental protection, and contains lipids and fatty acids to trap and retain moisture.

713 GET LIPPY

For an anti-ageing make-up effect, keep the eyes bare and wear a strong colour on the lips. This draws attention away from lines and wrinkles around the eyes and emphasizes the shape of the lips and lower jaw, giving a more youthful appearance.

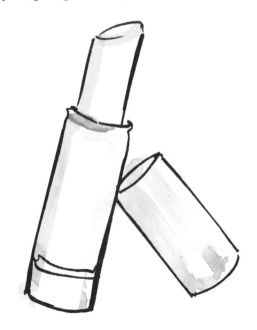

laser treatments

714 THERMO-TARGET YOUR VEINS

Thermo-coagulation is a vein-removal technique based on a high frequency wave producing a thermal lesion, which reduces the vein. A very fine needle is inserted into the vein, causing it to disappear instantaneously.

715 PULSE AWAY PIGMENT

With IPL (Intense Pulsed Light) technology, pulses of intense, concentrated light are directed onto the skin. These in turn are absorbed by the melanin in pigmented lesions such as age, sun and liver spots, which helps even out pigment problems.

716 RESURFACE YOUR SKIN

By delivering very powerful, rapid pulsing, the latest generation of CO_2 lasers removes fine lines and wrinkles of the face, smoothes acne scars, and rejuvenates ageing and sun-damaged skin as it contours the skin surface.

cosmetic fillers & treatments

717 CHECK THE CERTIFICATE

Make sure your therapist or nurse is properly trained and accredited. Ask to see copies of training certificates and if you're in any doubt, have them explain what their qualifications mean.

718 REST WITH RESTYLANE

Restylane injections involve plumping up facial lines and wrinkles by injecting small amounts of the filler into them, so they look plumper, smoother and softer.

719 PREPARE YOURSELF

If you're using a temporary filler cream at home, make sure your face is thoroughly cleansed and exfoliated so the filler can gloss over fine lines and form a smooth base for make-up. For salon-injected fillers, discuss any pre-care with your therapist beforehand.

720 DON'T GET CARRIED AWAY

When you're in the beauty room, it's tempting to want to look younger and younger, but you might regret going too far in the cold light of day! Take a photo of your youthful self into the treatment room so you can track just how much your appearance has changed – subtle is best.

721 SCULPT WITH SCULPTRA

Sculptra is a derivative of lactic acid, which aims to help do more than just fill in the wrinkle. It works from the inside out to stimulate the body's own production of collagen, making the skin appear smoother.

722 CALL ON COLLAGEN

Collagen appears less often now that Restylane and Perlane are common in salons, but it's still used for filling very fine lines on the brow and forehead and around the mouth. However, it does contain animal fats, so many vegetarians choose alternatives.

723 KNIT ONE, PERL ONE

Perlane is a filler made of the gel form of hyaluronic acid; it's a non-animal product whose effects last longer than traditional collagen because it affects the skin's mechanisms as well as filling the wrinkle. Because of this, it's a common choice for deeper lines and ageing skin.

724 GET FATTY

Another longer-lasting treatment for smoothing skin is autologous fat grafting, which uses fat extracted from one part of the body to "plump up" another part. It's also known as isolagen and the effect is more permanent than artificial products, so it's often used to combat sunken cheeks.

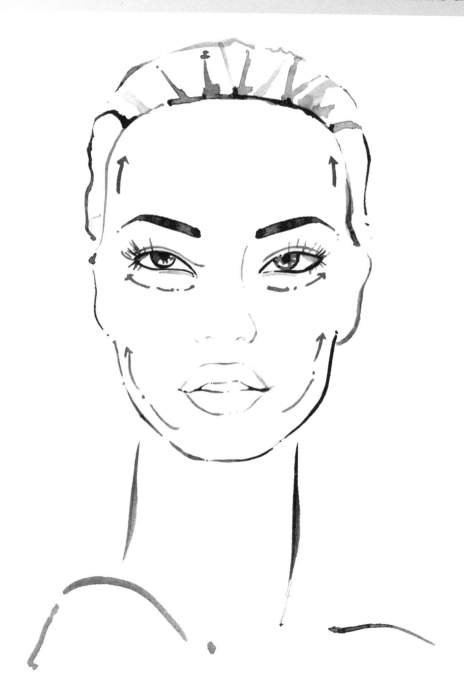

skin through the year

725 GO BALMY

The balmy summer nights might have long disappeared, but you can recapture some of that summer glow by choosing a balm instead of a cream or gel. Balms and oils are often a more effective way to reintroduce moisture to dehydrated skin.

726 GET SOME GOOD FATS

As your skin is exposed to winter elements, the natural oils are stripped away, especially in very windy weather. Choosing products with Essential Fatty Acids (EFAs) helps repair the skin's lipid layer to leave your skin protected, glowing and moisturized.

727 THINK AHEAD

If you've got dark hair and you want to be hair-free for summertime, consider starting your course of laser light therapy four to six months beforehand if you want the results to be visible, come swimwear season.

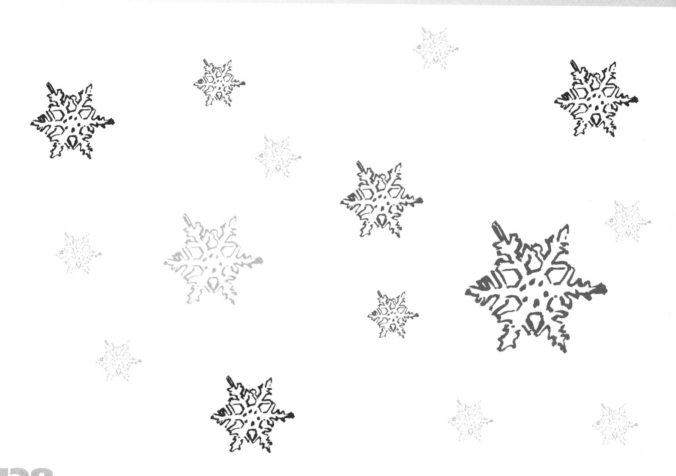

728 PERK UP WINTER SKIN

In extreme weather conditions cell renewal slows down, resulting in the skin thickening to protect itself and in the process becoming less vibrant. To stop your skin becoming flat and grey, use super-hydrating serums packed with hyaluronic acid to nourish and remoisturize.

729 KEEP OUT OF THE WIND

Strong winds are harmful as they cause moisture to evaporate, leaving skin dry, red and flaky. A skin cream that contains soy forms a protective barrier against the elements and gives intense hydration to dry and itchy skin.

730 TRY A TREATMENT MASK

Winter climates see a decline in the production of lipids (skin oils that seal in moisture). To compensate, use a revitalizing mask that contains a high amount of retinol to plump up fine lines and even out skin tone in more mature skin.

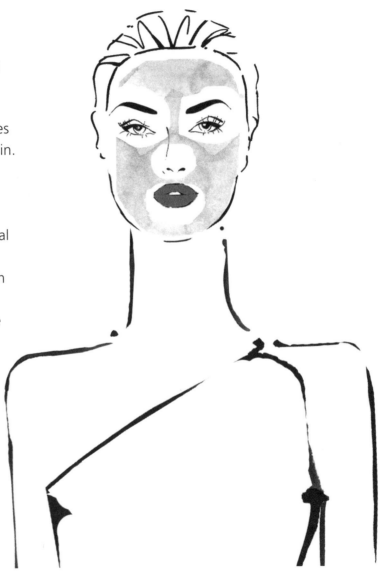

731 KEEP FABRICS SOFT

If your skin gets itchy during the winter, take a look at your fabrics – wearing abrasive fabrics such as wool and synthetic fibres next to the skin can cause dryness and itching, so try to make underlayers natural and soft.

732 STIR UP A SUMMER LOTION

Lotions (rather than creams) are a great choice for summer because they help lock moisture into the skin without blocking pores. Make your own by mixing equal amounts of glycerin, lime or lemon juice and rosewater, then apply half an hour before a bath to help give skin a moisture boost.

733 BE OATY

Give yourself a pre-bath winter vitamin and moisture boost by mixing a handful of oats with a tablespoon each of lime or lemon juice and milk. Apply to the whole body (but not the face), leave for 10 minutes and rinse before bathing.

734 TURN OFF THE HEAT

Winter skin suffers from too much time spent indoors in a dry atmosphere. Healthy skin has a water content of between 10 and 20 per cent, but central heating sucks natural moisture out to leave skin dry and dull-looking so lower the temperature of your heating and increase your intake of water.

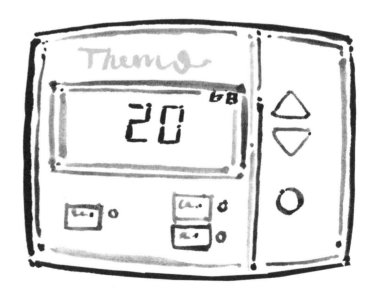

735 WISE UP TO WINTER

Harsh weather can lead to broken capillaries in the skin, caused by constant constricting and dilating of the blood vessels as you go from extreme cold outside to central heating inside. Increase your intake of vitamin C or use a serum containing high doses of it.

736 PLAN IN WINTER

Winter is the time to embark on cosmetic treatments requiring several weeks' or months' recovery, such as varicose veins and serious skin resurfacing. It's much easier to stay inside and out of the sun to recover than in summer, and you can keep areas covered up.

737 OVERNIGHT HYDRATION

While you are sleeping, the skin rests and repairs itself after the stresses of the day. At night, use a humidifier in your bedroom or place a damp towel over the radiator to replace moisture in the air and keep the skin hydrated. This helps to humidify the air around you, and reduces excessive water loss from the skin.

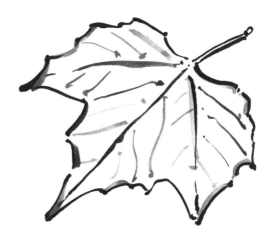

738 EXTREME WEATHER FLUSH

Travelling between cold exteriors and warm interiors can create a flushed red-faced complexion, straining blood vessels in the skin, which change size rapidly as the temperature fluctuates. Find a cream that contains peptides to help plump up skin so the broken veins don't show.

739 NIGHTY NIGHT!

During the winter months it's even more important to use a specially developed night cream to replace lost moisture while you sleep and protect against central heating dryness. Choose specialized products to look after winter skin.

740 LINE UP WITH VASELINE

Vaseline is a great choice for the care of dry skin as it helps coat the surface (and therefore it's unsuitable for oily or problem skin). Make up a winter body mask with equal amounts of Vaseline, glycerin and vitamin E oil for an all-over body moisturizing treatment. Wash off after an hour to let the skin breathe.

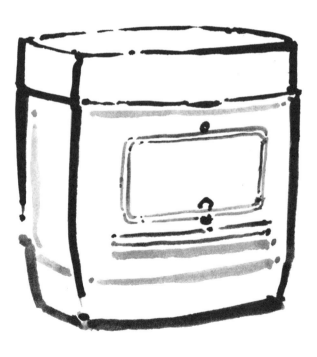

741 POLLUTION PROTECTION

Battle against polluted urban environments by using an SPF foundation or day cream specifically formulated to screen out the sun naturally with titanium dioxide, rather than one containing chemicals, which will contribute to the overload of toxins and environmental chemicals.

742 BE A BABY

Baby oil is a good choice for winter skin because it helps lock water onto the surface by providing a waterproof layer. After taking a bath, give your skin a watery treat by rubbing baby oil into wet skin. Leave it to dry naturally – don't rub it off with a towel.

743 HAVE A DRY SUMMER

Many people drink more when summer comes, but remember not only does the sun dry out your skin, but alcohol is also a dehydrating agent, which can lead to the skin becoming wrinkled and dry. Drink lots of water and avoid alcohol entirely several days a week.

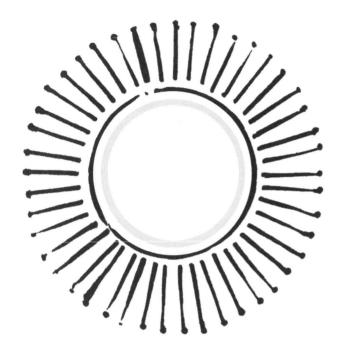

sun safety

744 CHECK YOUR REFLECTION

Don't assume that sitting in the shade of an umbrella or hat protects your skin adequately. Sunlight reflects from sand, snow, stone, wood and – particularly – water, so make sure you always protect yourself with sunscreen even if you're in the shade.

745 GO OFF-PEAK

Ninety per cent of problems associated with ageing are the result of too much sun exposure, so the best thing you can do to help your skin stay young is simply to avoid the sun. But because staying out of the sun entirely isn't an option for most people, aim to go off-peak. Avoid being in direct sunlight between 10 am and 4 pm – this is the most damaging time.

746 BE UV-FREE

If you're doing a lot of outside activity during the summer – like golf, sailing, gardening or walking – or if your job is outdoors, invest in some special UV screening clothing, particularly for your head and the top half of your body, which get the most exposure.

747 ADAPT YOUR ALTITUDE

The closer you are to the sun, the more powerful the sun's rays, and therefore the more damaging UV exposure you will suffer if you don't protect yourself. If you live, work or visit areas of high altitude, don't skimp on protection.

748 THE TWO-HOUR RULE

If you're in the sun, especially during the middle of the day, don't let two hours go by without reapplying your sunscreen – and you'll need to do this even more often if you're swimming or sweating a lot. You should use enough so that a thin layer sits on your skin before soaking in, rather than completely rubbing it in.

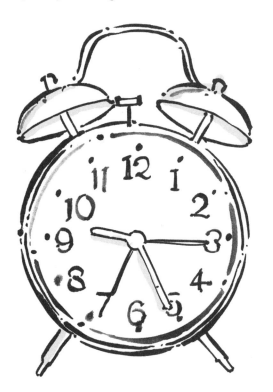

749 DON'T BE PSORALEN SORE

Some plant chemicals can increase the skin's sensitivity to UV light and this in turn increases your chances of sunburn and sun damage. Avoid psoralens (contained in citrus fruits, fennel, buttercups, cow parsley and celery) if you are prone to sun sensitivity.

750 CHECK YOUR INGREDIENTS

Retin-A, which is one of the most common drugs used in anti-acne treatments, and also in many anti-ageing face creams and products, can increase the skin's sensitivity to sunlight. Go carefully if you're a user, and always ask an expert for advice if you're at all concerned.

751 GET THE NUMBERS RIGHT

The way to choose the right sunscreen level is to first know the amount of time it would take for your skin to be in the sun before it burned, then multiply this figure by the SPF value. For instance, if you can expose your skin for 10 minutes before burning, an SPF 6 would prevent burning for 60 minutes, SPF 15 for 150 minutes and SPF 30 for 300 minutes.

752 ASK YOUR DOCTOR

Some antihistamines can make the skin more likely to burn with sun exposure – check with your doctor or nurse if you are taking antihistamines, antibiotics (tetracycline is one which can affect UV sensitivity) or NSAIDS.

753 AVOID THE BERGAMOT BURN

Bergamot is renowned for having some effect on the skin's ability to protect against sunlight. It's a common ingredient in bath and shower products because of its "citrus" smell, but if your skin is sensitive to sunlight or very pale, it might be worth giving it a miss for your morning shower.

754 SUP A SUPPLEMENT

Exposure to the sun requires different supplements to protect you against damage. Turmeric, an Indian root powder, has anti-inflammatory properties and is packed with antioxidants that can help combat the damage caused by UV exposure. Flax seed oil and fish oils provide a good dose of omega-3, while probiotics can also help reduce immune damage.

755 KEEP IT MATTE

Shiny, wet skin absorbs more light than dry skin because it enhances the way the rays of sunlight bend through liquids – that's why most tan accelerators are oil rather than cream based. Use creams for best protection.

sunscreens for all skin types

756 WEAR IT WELL

Concerned about sun exposure? Invest in a UV wristband – a disposable band you wear on your wrist for the day, which measures sun exposure and turns red when you've had enough.

757 NOT TOO HASTY

To make sure that you get the most out of your sunscreen, allow 15 to 30 minutes for any moisturizer to soak into the skin before applying. This will ensure the sunblock works correctly.

758 GO IMMORTAL

One of the best natural products to protect against sun damage and UV penetration is a plant called statice, also known as "*immortelle bleue*" in France, its country of origin. A powerful antioxidant, when used as a skin preparation or supplement, statice can help regulate sun exposure to reduce damage.

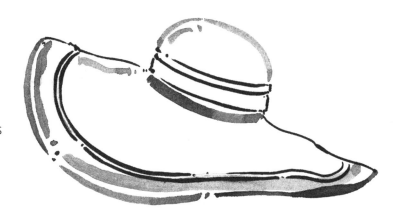

759 GO OVER-30

Always aim to use a sunscreen of factor 30 or more, especially if you are in the sun during the middle of the day, or for longer than a few hours. And remember SPFs don't add up – applying factor 15 twice doesn't give you more protection, just a thicker layer!

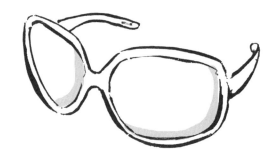

760 GET THE RIGHT DOSAGE

For a sunscreen to live up to its SPF rating, 2 mg should be applied for every square centimetre of exposed skin, which means on average you should be using 100 mg for every four whole body applications. Most people don't use anything like enough.

761 WEAR A HAT

The best way to protect the skin on your face while in the sun is to wear a cream with a minimum SPF 15, plus a hat to shade your face to make sure no damaging rays get through. Sunglasses protect the delicate eye area, but a wide-brimmed hat will cover the whole lot.

762 ALL MADE UP

For best results, apply make-up first and then pat sunblock over the top to ensure even protection against the sun. This also prevents your make-up sliding down your face when you're trying to look glamorous on the beach!

763 GET PROTECTED

A day cream with SPF is a great choice, but they're not intended for sun exposure. Use a dedicated sun cream if you're going to be spending time outside. If you don't like the greasy feel, instead of applying sun cream with fingers, try using a sponge to help the cream really penetrate the skin while making sure you apply a thick enough layer for protection.

764 PACK A SERUM PUNCH

Serums contain powerful ingredients in high concentrations, which your face will need if it's taking an unaccustomed sun, sand and sea battering. For holiday skin, look for serums containing antioxidants such as vitamins A, C and E for great results.

765 LIKE IT LIGHT

If your skin is prone to acne or breakouts, it's worth choosing a lighter, non-occlusive sunscreen with chemical blocks such as avobenzone, oxybenzone, methoxycinnamate or octocrylene. Mineral blocks like zinc oxide and titanium oxide tend to sit on top of the skin, which can aggravate acne and breakouts.

766 ANNUAL CULL

After a year, sunscreen loses its protective ability so when summer comes to a close, throw away any leftover sunscreen so you're not tempted to re-use it the next year.

767 GO GENTLY

If you find your skin reacts to sunscreens and becomes red, sore or blotchy, this might be due to chemical sunblocks such as oxybenzone, which have been thought to cause reactions in some people with sensitive skin. Choose a mineral block sunscreen instead of chemical – check the ingredients list carefully.

768 JOIN THE CLUB

It's not only those with fair skin who need protection against sun exposure. Damage to dark skins can be harder to spot early on, so it's even more important to get covered. Choose an SPF of at least 8, but preferably 15, or even 30 for prolonged exposure.

holiday skin

769 TAKE A TRIMMER

If you're holidaying for more than a week, your bikini line is likely to need attention while you're away. Take along a bikini trimmer to target the areas you don't want to shave – make sure you remember your adapter plug for rechargeable items.

770 SINK IN THE SAND

One of the most useful substances you'll find on your summer holiday is sand. When damp from the sea, sand is the perfect way to exfoliate without using chemicals. Simply lie or sit at the water's edge and gently scrub a handful into your skin, brushing up toward your heart. Plunge hands into the sand and walk on damp sand to exfoliate feet.

771 GO LOCAL

If you're holidaying somewhere hot and by the sea, take advantage of the local diet, which is likely to be high in all the right foods to help protect you against the damage caused by exposure to the sun and the elements. Look especially for fish, fruit, vegetables and local combinations of spices.

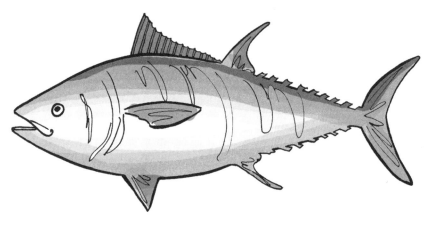

772 ENJOY A BALMY NIGHT

One essential product you should pack for your holiday in the sun is a glycerin-based balm, which helps calm and rehydrate your face if you take the sunbathing a bit too far, or your skin starts to react to being covered with sun cream.

773 WRAP UP SOME WEED

Seaweed is an excellent choice for super-hydrated, nourished skin, being packed full of vitamins and minerals, and because the structure is so similar to skin, it's easily absorbed. For a simplest spa treatment of all, cover yourself in seaweed and lie in the shallow sea for 10 minutes.

774 TAKE A DIP

Seawater has long been thought to hold health benefits as it's not just salty but stacked full of minerals, which can help calm skin conditions and boost the immune system. Take a dip to expose your skin to the seawater – aim to stay in for at least 10 minutes.

775 CORRECT DARK SPOTS

Another great choice for holiday skin is a dark spot corrector containing whitening or pigment balancing agents. Freckles might make you look sun-kissed, but larger pigment spots can be unsightly so having something with you to help begin the correction process gives you a good start.

776 USE AN OIL

Summer skin is often more dehydrated and dry, especially if you are holidaying in the sun of a colder, more humid climate. Using a face oil every night on vacation will give your skin a chance to recover as you sleep and also reduces the amount of damage inflicted on it while you're away.

777 BOOK YOURSELF A TREATMENT

At the same time as you book your pre-summer holiday treatments such as leg waxing or hair colouring, book yourself in for a post-holiday facial treatment to eliminate any remaining sun damage or dehydration. A week after you get back home is ideal.

778 GO WATERPROOF

Understanding the difference between water resistant and waterproof could be the difference between tanning and burning, especially if your holiday involves swimming or watersports. Water-resistant sunscreen is designed to last 30 to 40 minutes in the water (waterproof 80 to 90 minutes).

spotting & treating sun damage

779 E FOR EFFECTIVE

The single best ingredient in creams, lotions and oils to help reduce and prevent sun damage from taking a lasting hold on skin is vitamin E. It is present in many after-sun lotions but choose a concentrated version to ensure your skin doesn't suffer because of your sun-soaking habit.

780 TOWEL DOWN

If you burn the skin on your face, soak the damaged area in cool water or place a damp, cold flannel over it for 10 minutes to take away redness and swelling. Avoid alcohol, smoke and further sun until the redness fades, and use moisturizer twice a day.

781 COVER YOUR MOLES

If you have lots of moles, it's a sign that your skin is more sensitive to the sun than others – the guidelines on reducing sun exposure are especially important for you to follow. Make sure you constantly cover moles with a high-factor sunscreen, too.

782 OATY TREAT

Fill a sock or stocking with oatmeal and hang it under the tap (faucet) as you run a bath so the water flows through it. Remove the bag before you bathe, and try to stay in the water for at least 10 minutes. This is a good remedy for a whole range of skin complaints, from dermatitis and eczema to nettle rash and sunburn.

783 COOL DOWN SUMMER BURN

Chlorine, sun and high temperatures can make the skin on your legs more prone to post-shave stinging and rashes. Use a lotion with Aloe to soothe – store it in the refrigerator for 20 minutes before use for a soothing treat that will really cool skin.

784 MEDICATE YOUR MOISTURIZER

To a plain, unscented moisturizer, add a few drops of aloe and tea tree oil. Apply liberally over areas affected by sunburn. If you suffer a lot, make up a bottle of this home-made concoction and keep it by your bed to use whenever you feel sore or tight.

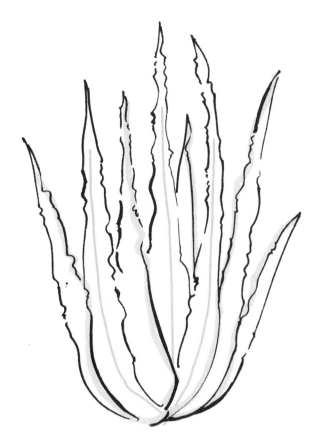

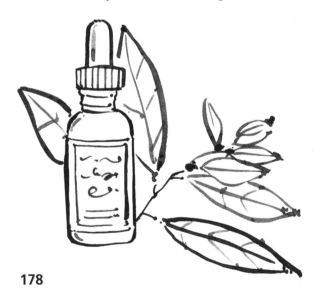

785 SOOTHE SUNBURN

Ease those sunburnt areas and prevent itching, soreness and further damage with a lotion of half a cup of witch hazel mixed with a quarter of a cup each of aloe vera gel, baby oil and high-factor sunscreen.

786 MAKE A PACT

If you notice any changes on your skin and are worried about them, seek medical advice immediately, especially if the change has taken place over a few months, rather than years. Why not make a pact with a friend or partner to check each other's skin once every month for any changes? The more often you look, the more likely you are to spot anything new.

787 REMEMBER YOUR LEGS

Don't forget your lower legs when you're in the sun – it's the most common site for skin cancer in women as they often forget they're exposed. Be sure to include them in your daily SPF protection.

788 BATHE IN VINEGAR

To treat sunburn, add a cup of cider or white vinegar to a bath of lukewarm or cool water and sit in it for as long as you feel comfortable. This will help reduce redness and soreness of the skin. Pat dry carefully and apply a cooling moisturizer.

maintain a healthy glow

789 START RIGHT

Self-tanners contain a chemical called DHA, which stains the uppermost layer of skin, so it's better to get the product right in the first place than to try and correct any mistakes. Don't skimp on preparation – and that means making your skin "palate" smooth, clear and well hydrated.

790 LAYER UP FOR A SMOOTH TAN

Perfect the no-streaks, natural-looking tan with a little patience! Instead of slathering it all on at once, apply a little self-tan at a time and build up the colour with a second application a few days later.

791 GO EASY ON DRY SKIN

Dry skin around the knees, elbows and ankles picks up self-tan colour more. Instead of applying tan neat, mix with moisturizer to avoid dark patches on these areas.

782 EXFOLIATE DAILY

Prepare your skin for self-tanning by exfoliating daily for the three or four days before you apply it. Following exfoliation, use moisturizer liberally to build up smoothness and hydration in the skin and prevent uneven streaks. Before any kind of tanning session, shower and exfoliate first and use cleanser instead of soap to keep the skin's moisture levels high.

783 BLOT AND BRONZE

Before applying bronzer, blot your skin with blotting papers or a clean tissue – this gives the skin an even surface and ensures blotch-free bronzer.

794 SHAVE OFF SKIN

Shaving not only removes hairs, it also serves to exfoliate the skin so it's a great hair-removal choice at least 12 hours before you apply self-tan. Avoid shaving for a day or two afterwards, though, as it could weaken the tan or cause streaks. If waxing, aim for 24 hours in advance as it's inadvisable to apply tanner to red, inflamed or irritated skin.

785 HIDE THE MARK

If tan lines caused by bikinis, skimpy tops, shorts and socks are blighting your quest for an all-over tan, smooth out marks by applying small amounts of fake tan (mix with moisturizer first so you don't go too dark). For an even-looking colour, simply reapply as tan fades.

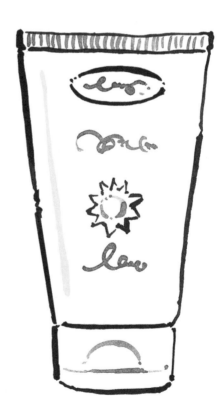

786 GO EASY ON THE MOISTURIZER

Although dry skin is a tanning no-no, too much moisturizer is one of the biggest fake tan mistakes because it creates a barrier between the skin and the tan, making it more prone to slipping and streaks. Always wait until the cream has soaked in before applying fake tan.

787 LAYER UP WITH LATEX

To avoid the telltale "orange hands" of the at-home fake tanner, invest in a box of Latex gloves to protect dry areas on palms from accumulating product. After applying elsewhere on the body, use the gloves to apply a small amount to the back of your hands before discarding them.

788 MIX IT UP

It's rare for natural tans to be completely even and, with a bit of practice, you can mirror this effect with fake tan. Make the tan slightly stronger on the fronts and backs of legs by layering up product, and mix self tanner with moisturizer for feet, ankles, knees and elbows.

799 SPATULA IT ON

If you're applying fake tan to your skin but there's no one to do your back for you, invest in a back-tanning spatula to reach those hard-to-get-to areas so you don't miss a bit!

800 VAS UP YOUR HAIRLINE

To avoid fake tan accumulating around hair and hairlines, use a small smear of Vaseline to cover eyebrows and hairline and prevent product build-up.

801 TAKE PRECAUTIONS

If you choose to use a tanning bed, make sure your eyes and lips are protected, and cover any moles with sunblock. Also, check with your doctor first: certain medications can react with UV exposure.

802 BUFF IT UP

A buffing mitt is a great way to make sure that your tan isn't streaky or uneven. Use it to gently disperse any areas where you have noticed product build-up, to give a more even appearance.

803 DON'T BE TIGHT

The best possible thing to do after a fake tan is to wear nothing for a while to avoid patches developing, but that's not always possible. Do choose loose-fitting, dark clothes, though and avoid tight lines and getting too much material in contact with the skin.

804 RUB IT OUT

Don't panic if your self-tan goes wrong, or if it makes your skin too dark – self-tan remover is a great way to remove any unwanted dye from the skin, returning your skin to a more natural shade.

805 PROLONG YOUR TAN

One of the best ways to extend the life of your fake tan is to gently exfoliate and thoroughly moisturize daily. If you do this evenly, your tan should fade without patches and you can top up when it starts to get too pale.

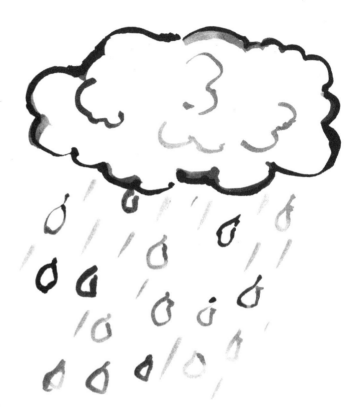

806 DON'T GET WET

Water is a nightmare for self-tanners – avoid washing up, washing your hands, showering, bathing, going out in the rain and anything else involving water for at least eight hours after application. Where possible, apply last thing at night.

hair removal

807 GO AGAINST THE GRAIN

Unlike when men shave their faces, body hair removal requires movement against the growth of the hair for best results – which means working up your leg from ankle to knee and bikini line, then underarms from inside up and out.

808 STIFFEN UP

If you're really inflexible but you're going for a bikini waxing appointment, let the therapist know beforehand so they won't expect you to be able to get into positions you find uncomfortable. Similarly, tell them about injuries, bruises and areas of soreness for a range of treatments.

809 BE CLEAN

Any hair removal technique that involves pulling the hair out from the root – that is plucking, waxing (at home or in the salon) and epilating – works best when skin is clean. Drier skin is smoother, so wash and dry thoroughly, unless you are wet epilating.

810 KNOW YOUR TRIM

Many salons seem to call different bikini waxes by different names but the general consensus is that the "Brazilian" is mostly trimmed except for a strip at the front, while the "Hollywood" means all the hair is removed. Knowing what to ask for is key if you want to get the right look.

811 LASER AWAY HAIRS

IPL, or Intense Pulsed Light, is a great choice for hair removal as well as acne scarring, sun damage and fine lines. In many beauty salons, it has largely replaced electrolysis. Be careful, though: it only works to remove hair if your hair and skin are recognizably different colours so it's not a good choice for fair, red, grey or white hair.

812 TRIM AWAY

If you're using a home epilator, the most effective and comfortable way to do this is to buy a wet and dry device because the water soothes skin. To minimize discomfort, make sure hair is 2 to 3 mm long (most come with a trimmer).

813 STRETCH IT OUT

As you get older, your skin grows less elastic and bikini waxing can become more painful and traumatic to skin. Stretching the skin is a great way to minimize pain and trauma – let your therapist know at the beginning of the session that you are happy to help with the stretch and follow their instructions.

814 WASH AND BRUSH UP

After using a home epilator or shaver, make sure you wash the blades or epilator head thoroughly each time by running underwater to wash away hairs, then dry carefully. If hairs stick to the blades, use an old toothbrush or special cleaning brush to carefully brush them away.

815 DON'T SHARE

If you're using a home hair removal device such as a lady shave or a home epilator, make sure you rinse the head before applying to different parts of your body to avoid transferring bacteria. And never share equipment, even with close family members.

816 GO SILVER

Look for an epilator with both tweezers and discs, which will remove hair of different lengths and thicknesses; also adjustable heads for quicker results. Silver coating reduces bacterial build-up, too.

817 WEEKLY DOES IT

If you're new to epilating, it's best to epilate once a week for the first three weeks to allow your skin to get used to the sensation. This also ensures you remove all the hairs which are growing in different cycles.

818 TRY TURMERIC

The best natural depilator is a turmeric paste, which gets rid of even thick hairs. For a naturally smooth look, apply before a bath, leave to dry and then simply wash off.

819 BE A NIGHT OWL

When epilating or waxing at home, doing it at night is a good choice because that way the skin can calm down and repair any small amount of damage overnight.

820 BE GENTLE

Home shaving and epilation require a gentle touch. Today's machinery is designed to work with only gentle pressure, so pushing into the skin can cause discomfort and prevent it from working as it should.

821 BLEACH AWAY DOWN

If you have downy hair on your forehead or in front of your ears, rub a freshly cut lemon over the hair. Leave for five to 10 minutes before rinsing off – it's a natural bleaching agent which won't make them bright white.

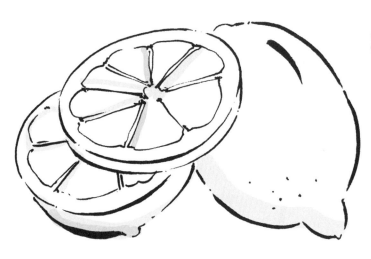

822 HOLD IT STRAIGHT

For the most effective home epilation, make sure your epilator is held straight against the skin at 90 degrees, so the hairs don't pull. Use your other hand to stretch skin to facilitate hair removal. The same applies for lady shavers, which are designed for straight-on use.

823 WAX AWAY

When waxing at home, make sure you apply wax in the direction of hair growth, then pull it out away from that direction to avoid breaking hair off at the root.

824 TIME OF THE MONTH

In the few days before your period, when hormone levels in the body are out of balance, waxing can be more painful. Check your diary before you de-fuzz. If you find the pain of waxing or epilating too much to bear, lessen it by taking an aspirin or paracetamol 15 minutes beforehand.

825 STAY COOL

Cooler skin is more responsive to light, so if you're using laser therapy you should avoid bathing or showering in warm water for half an hour before your treatment.

826 WARM UP INGROWING HAIRS

To treat ingrown pubic hairs along the bikini line, hold a hot compress against ingrown spots for 10 minutes a couple of times a day. It softens skin and help the hairs work their way out.

827 DON'T RUB RED SPOTS

If you have red spots caused by ingrowing hairs or sore patches following hair removal on your bikini line, wear loose-fitting underwear and clothing until the bumps are gone to avoid friction. Avoid the temptation to pick at spots, too.

828 SAY ALOE FOR SENSITIVE SKIN

If your skin is sensitive, choose a razor with an added aloe vera strip to lubricate and soothe as you shave. It also prevents pulling and decreases the chances of irritation.

829 GET IN A LATHER

You don't have to use special shaving foam in order to get a close shave – shampoo is a great choice as it creates a stiffer lather than body wash, or use conditioner for more slippery shaving.

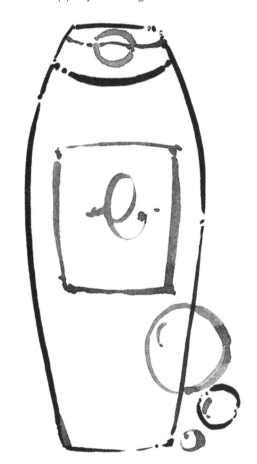

830 BE A WATER BABY

To ensure an extremely close shave, soften hairs first by taking a short, warm bath – hair is easier to cut when wet and supple. But don't soak in the bath for too long or run the water too hot, as this causes skin to wrinkle and swell.

831 GET THE SLANT

When plucking areas such as the brows, chin or upper lip, choose slanted or angled tweezers for targeted hair removal. The slant makes it easier to grasp and pluck in the direction of hair growth, which in turn reduces soreness and redness.

832 AVOID OILS

If you're using a home epilator, covering your legs with foam or wash is a good idea as it can make the process more comfortable and smoother. Avoid any product containing an essential oil, however, as these can prevent the hair being properly gripped.

833 RUB IT UP

For the best results from your wax or epilation session, spend a minute or so rubbing all over the area to be treated with the palms of your hands beforehand. This makes the hairs stand away from the skin for more effective results.

834 DON'T WAX SUNBURN

Laser peels and sunburn are two big no-nos when it comes to waxing. Because they expose the more sensitive layers of the skin and can cause redness and heat retention in skin layers, you should avoid waxing within a week of either.

835 GO FLAT FOR LARGE

For large areas of hair removal – for example, touching up patches on legs or arms that may have been missed with waxing – use flat-headed tweezers or a home epilator. This pulls out more than one hair at a time and makes plucking more efficient.

836 BEWARE OF WAXING

If you are using Retin-A, Accutane or other skin-exfoliating medications, tell your beautician before your waxing appointment as increased skin sensitivity can occur. They might even want to change your treatment.

837 GO EASY WITH CAMOMILE

Many spas use camomile wax – regular wax infused with calming camomile, which can ease the pain and redness that often occurs following waxing. If you have sensitive skin, seek advice from your beautician.

838 BE A SUGAR, SUGAR

Sugaring is frequently a better choice than waxing if you've got somewhere to go afterwards, as wax can stick to legs but the sugar solution is water soluble, which means it wipes off, leaving no telltale marks.

839 GET TRIM

Trimming hair with nail scissors before bikini waxing makes the job a lot easier as it prevents tangles and can reduce pain. You'll get straight lines too and avoid that uneven look.

840 TREAT FACIAL HAIR WITH ROSE

Stimulating facial hair will cause it to grow more. To avoid this, use a light toner such as rosewater and a light moisturizer that won't nourish the hair roots.

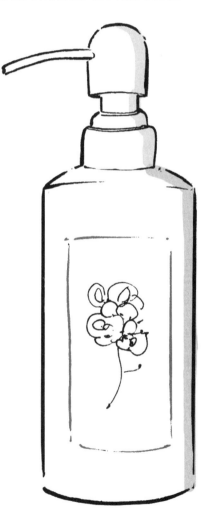

841 EXFOLIATE BEFORE YOU WAX

To avoid ingrowing hairs post-waxing, remove dead skin cells that could obstruct the hairs beforehand by exfoliating the area to be waxed first. Because skin will be softer, you are less likely to develop ingrowing hairs.

842 KEEP IT COOL

Avoid saunas, hot baths, exercise or sunbathing for 24 hours after hair removal. All of these can raise your body temperature, which means you may sweat more and cause irritation to treated areas.

coping with chemicals, salt & chlorine

843 AVOID REACTIVE SKIN

Use a cream with a mild hydrocortisone included for problem skin that's prone to rashes and redness. The anti-inflammatory products will help your skin maintain a healthy profile.

844 RINSE WELL

Salt water, especially naturally salty seawater, has many benefits for the skin but leaving it on can cause skin to become dry and itchy. Help your skin get the benefits without dehydration by rinsing off after each dip with a cool, fresh water shower.

845 BE A CHEMIST

If you're spending a lot of time in chlorinated water, your skin and hair will benefit from a specifically designed chemically rebalancing wash. Some companies even make washes intended for specific chemical levels so do your research before you buy.

846 SAY ALOE

If your skin is sensitive to chlorine, and especially if it becomes red and dry a few hours after your swim, choose products to help soothe it once you're out of the water. For example, products containing aloe vera will gently cleanse and also reduce inflammation.

PROBLEM SKIN

sensitive skin secrets

847 SCENT SENSITIVITY

Instead of using a scented sunscreen on sensitive skin, opt for an unscented alternative containing organic, plant-based ingredients, such as aloe vera, jojoba, avocado and camomile.

848 DON'T GO MICRO

Microdermabrasion is a great choice for deep exfoliation and, because it takes off the top few layers of skin, it can help reduce fine lines, large pores and pigmentation. Be careful if you have sensitivity, redness or problem skin as it can cause some conditions to become worse, though.

849 KEEP IT SIMPLE

When it comes to sensitive skin, less is definitely more. Aim to limit the products you use to just a few tried-and-tested favourites – challenging sensitive skin with new products can make it more prone to reaction.

850 START GENTLY

When looking for a cleanser to suit your sensitive skin, it's all about balance – you want to find the mildest cleanser which works without having to rub your skin too hard, or wash your face more than once to remove make-up and dirt. Start gently and work your way up.

851 MSM RULES

The supplementary form of sulphur in the diet – MSM – has been shown to help reduce skin problems such as sensitivity, dryness, eczema and psoriasis. Although present in lots of raw vegetables, fruit, milk, eggs and fish, sulphur is often lost during the cooking process so consider taking a supplement.

852 DON'T BE ANTI-MICROBIAL

Many people use anti-microbial products such as hand soap but don't be tempted to apply them to your face – often they contain harsh chemicals that can dry out skin and cause reactions.

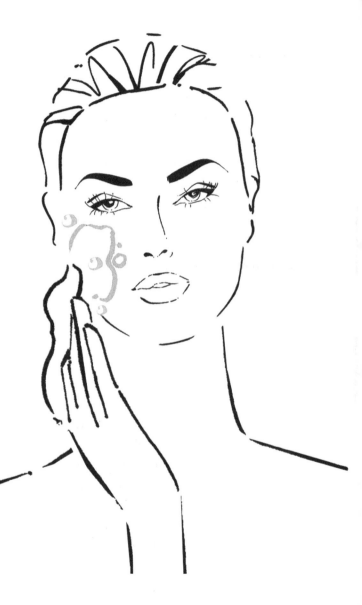

853 GO MINERAL

If you find your skin reacts to sunscreen, the chances are you're reacting to oxybenzone. Most sunscreens now no longer contain PABA (Para-aminobenzoic acid) as it has caused so many reactions, but instead choose mineral sunscreens, such as zinc oxide and titanium oxide and be sure to cleanse well at night.

854 GO FRAGRANCE-FREE

Just because a product is natural or derived from an essential oil or plant product doesn't mean it can't cause sensitive skin to react and repeated exposure only makes matters worse. Watch out for cinnamon, camphor, eucalyptus, fragrance, menthol, lavender, rosewater and peppermint on labels.

simple first-aid tips

855 MAKE A REMEDY

Make your own skin-healing solution by picking the flowers from St John's Wort and infuse in a bottle of extra virgin olive oil or almond oil. Leave out in the sun every day for a few hours until the oil turns a deep brown (this could be weeks or months, depending on sun strength) and then store in a cool, dark place. Use as a topical treatment for bites, stings, bruises and other minor skin problems.

856 HEAVEN CENT

Centella asiatica – an Indian/Sri Lankan herb also known as Gotu kola – has been shown to help skin to repair by enhancing the structures deep inside which support collagen and promote blood flow. Take 100 mg daily, split into two or three doses, and look for a version containing 70 per cent of the active ingredients triterpenoids.

857 ASK FOR ALOE

Aloe is a great healer for all skin problems, but it's especially good for burns because of its nourishing, hydrating and cooling powers. The best way to use it is to cut fresh leaves and apply the juice direct to the skin, but a tube of aloe vera gel could also be used.

858 SUPPLEMENT YOUR HEALING

The single most important thing the skin needs for wound healing is collagen and to produce adequate supplies the body needs vitamins C, B, A, E and zinc, so make sure if you have suffered a wound (especially if you have other parts of your body that need repairing, too) that you take a supplement or up their intake in your diet.

859 GET OIL-E

For wounds that do not break the skin, such as bruises, blisters and burns, vitamin E oil is a great choice because it helps promote skin healing but doesn't block pores or cause infection. Because of this it helps speed up the healing process, but also reduces the formation of scar tissue.

860 SIT ON THE DOCK

If you suffer a nettle sting, look around for nature's own remedy – dock leaves are flat, green leaves that are usually found growing side by side with nettles but whose leaves contain a remedy for the irritating sting. Mash up a leaf between your fingers until the juice runs and apply to the sting.

861 BE COMFY WITH COMFREY

Comfrey has great healing properties, especially for swollen or inflamed skin. Use the leaves as a poultice for insect bites and stings, pound the leaves into a paste to apply to minor burns and scalds, and soak the root in your bath to refresh skin.

862 REMEMBER RICE

The single most effective thing you can do for any type of injury is to use the RICE technique – Rest, Ice, Compression and Elevation – and skin injuries are no different. Pressing ice onto an affected area is the best way to reduce inflammation, pain and itching.

863 GET A NATURAL CURE

Many natural substances have the power to reduce inflammation and itching after bites and stings – look for those with natural antiseptic or anti-inflammatory properties, such as witch hazel, lavender, tea tree, calamine and manuka honey.

864 STOP SQUEEZING

If a sting is sticking in the skin, avoid squeezing it – even if this does remove the sting, it could cause more of the irritating chemical to enter. Instead, use a sharp edge, such as a fingernail, ruler or credit card, to scrape the sting away.

865 GET COLD

If you suffer a burn, the best thing to do is immediately plunge the area into cold (preferably iced) water or hold it under a running cold tap. Leave it there for as long as possible until the heat has left the skin.

866 SWAB WITH TEABAGS

Use warm (not hot), used teabags for swabbing minor cuts, grazes and swelling. Tea contains natural antioxidants and anti-inflammatories.

scarring

867 MAKE A BIO CHOICE

Bio-oil, which contains the active ingredient PurCellin oil to specifically target scars and reduce their colour and shape, also contains vitamins A and E and essential oils to further strengthen skin. Apply daily.

868 HOPE FOR HYALURONIC

In some trials hyaluronic acid has been shown to assist in the healing of wounds by maximizing the potential to heal and renew. Never use on broken skin, where there is a risk of infection, but apply creams containing this ingredient whenever your skin needs a helping hand.

869 SUGAR AND SPICE

Honey and nutmeg can be used to reduce and soften scars. Combine a teaspoon of nutmeg (freshly grated works best) with a teaspoon of honey. Apply to the scarred area and leave it there for 15 minutes, then wash off. For best results, use a few times a week.

870 BUY A PAPAYA

The inside of papaya skin can be used to help reduce scarring as it contains enzymes and compounds which help the skin to heal itself naturally; it also assists in the treatment of spots and blemishes. Wipe the inside of a papaya skin over your face, leave for an hour and wash off with warm water.

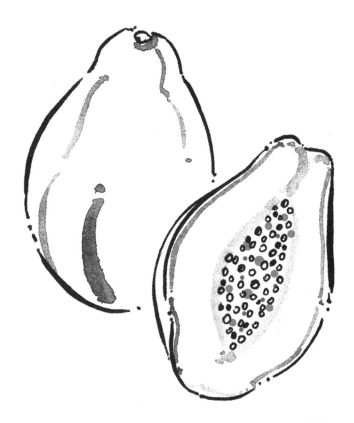

871 GET SOUR

Finely chop an onion and use a muslin or strainer to extract the juice, or use a juicer. Mix one part onion juice with one part cider vinegar and apply the formulation directly onto scarred or discolored areas of skin.

872 COOL AS A CUCUMBER

Applying fresh cucumber juice can help reduce scarring as it maintains the right fluid balance in the skin, which helps it heal more effectively. Juice a cucumber and use as a lotion, or lie still with fresh cucumber slices placed over the affected areas for 10 minutes a day.

873 WEAR SANDALS WITH PRIDE

Sandalwood paste can help remove scarring, particularly scars left by acne or other skin conditions. Make a paste by rubbing a sandalwood stick on a wooden board with some rosewater, then use as a face pack for 5 to 10 minutes before rinsing.

874 SMEAR ON SOME HONEY

If you are worried about scarring, try smearing honey over the affected area – it is thought to help the skin cells bind together, reducing the appearance of scars by speeding up the healing process. Manuka honey is the best to choose for this process because of its powerful antiseptic properties.

875 FRESHEN UP ACNE SCARS

Crush up a handful of mint leaves and wrap in a piece of muslin cloth. Squeeze and roll to extract the juice, then wipe the bag all over your face using gentle circular movements. Do this daily to help reduce acne scarring.

876 BE A HIPPY

Rosehip can help heal scarring and reverse skin discoloration. Simply cut a rosehip in half and wipe over the scar, or make a rosehip tea to use as a refreshing facial rinse following cleansing.

rosacea

877 SPICE ISN'T NICE

Rosacea can be exacerbated by foods containing chilli and mustard, and by hot drinks, which cause an increase in circulation and can make redness worse. Skin also feels hot and uncomfortable.

878 GO FOR THE BURN

Chilli might not seem an obvious choice for sore skin but the capsaicin it contains can help relieve pain and itching by blocking nerves. Add half a teaspoon of cayenne pepper to your usual moisturizing cream or oil, but test a small area first to check for stinging, and keep away from eyes and lips.

879 OWN UP

If you suffer from rosacea, there's no need to hide it – this condition affects as many as one in 20 people, and about three times as many of these are women than men. Don't worry about feeling a bit flushed, or be ashamed or embarrassed about it as this actually exacerbates the condition.

880 UP YOUR ACIDS

If you suffer from rosacea and also have heartburn, indigestion and feelings of fullness, bloating or bad breath, you may be suffering from low levels of stomach acid or of the digestive enzyme lipase. A nutritionist or doctor will help you choose the right supplement.

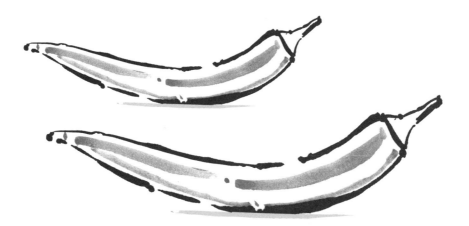

881 COVER UP

Rosacea most commonly occurs on the face, particularly on the cheeks of those who have fair hair. If you are a sufferer, try to avoid exposing your cheeks to harsh weather conditions, such as hail, snow, strong sunshine, rain or extreme cold. Using a scarf to cover your face if you're outside in these conditions can help prevent redness.

882 GO ALOE

Aloe vera is a great substance for soothing the skin without causing dryness as it nourishes, as well as cools. It's a great choice for applying to skin beneath tinted moisturizer or foundation as it can help prevent redness from showing through.

883 GREEN IS GOOD

When it comes to skincare, green and red are at opposite ends of the spectrum so if your cheeks appear really red, try using a colour corrective stick underneath your make-up to help level out your skintone. Be careful not to over-use, though – less is more!

884 FIND THE TRIGGER

Although there are well-known suspects, everyone with rosacea is likely to have a slightly different trigger. Keep a food diary for several weeks to try and work out what makes your rosacea worse and remove or cut down on those ingredients in your diet.

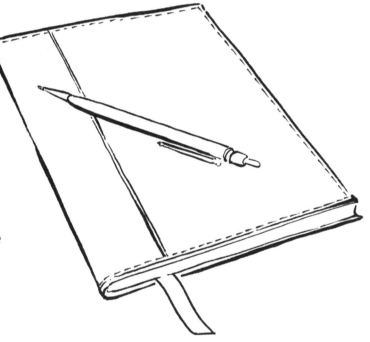

885 TRY SHORT-TERM STEROIDS

Topical steroids can be used on a short-term basis to help reduce the symptoms of rosacea. However, long-term use could actually make the condition worse because it thins the skin and may cause additional problems.

886 NOT SO HARSH

If you suffer from rosacea, you should at all times avoid astringents and harsh soaps. Not only can they make the symptoms worse, they also dry out skin, making it harder to treat and cover.

887 DRY OUT

Avoid alcohol as this increases blood flow to the face, which can cause an increase in redness. It also dehydrates, which may make skin appear dryer. The same goes for extremes of temperature, which can have the same effect.

888 B HIGH

If you suffer rosacea, make sure you supplement daily with a high potency B-vitamin complex. Find one that contains at least 100 mg of each of the B-vitamins to help promote the most effective reduction in inflammation and the best skin healing.

acne

889 TEA FOR TWO?

One of the best natural anti-acne treatments is tea tree oil, derived from the Australian plant *Melaleuca alternifolia*, or tea tree. It's a great way to help reduce inflammation and infection in the skin without the side effects of chemical treatments. Choose creams or oils with added tea tree oil rather than using it neat.

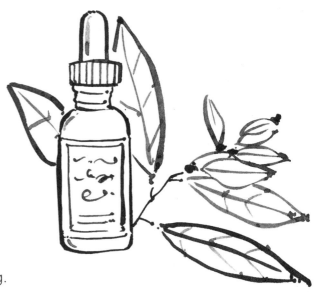

890 STICK IT TO THEM

After using brushes or concealer sticks to cover up blemishes or spots, always wash them well to avoid re-infection. Or use cotton buds, which are disposable.

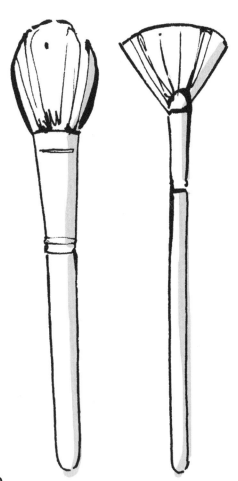

891 GET SILVER

Silverweed (*Potentilla anserina*) is a flowering plant that is thought to have some calming and antiseptic qualities. Pound the yellow flowers to a pulp and use as a topical treatment for spots, provided that the skin isn't broken.

892 TAKE A TONIC

Make your own witch-hazel astringent to treat spots, cuts, blackheads and oily areas of skin. Combine one cup of witch hazel with two tablespoons ethanol alcohol and apply to your skin with a cotton ball. If you want to be alcohol-free, use clear vinegar instead.

893 DITCH THE HABIT

If you have spotty or oily skin, keep your hands away from your face and pay particular attention to habits like rubbing the temples or around the mouth, which you may do subconsciously. Ask a friend or partner to help you watch out for this.

884 HOLD THE SCRUB

Beware of over-exfoliating spotty or oily areas of the skin. On problem skin, exfoliation can cause excess oils to be released, making the problem worse and it can cause acne to spread to uninfected areas. Instead use gentle polishers to treat oily areas only.

885 GET A DIAGNOSIS

If you are a women who has developed acne later in life, in your twenties, thirties or beyond, check with your doctor that you're not suffering PCOS (Polycystic Ovary Syndrome), which is a common cause. Ask to change your pill because acne in women is often hormonal.

886 PREVENT SPREAD

If you're worried about infection from acne eruptions spreading to other parts of your face, use a topical antibiotic to contain the infection. Never squeeze, as it could make the pores swell further and look worse and avoid metal extractor tools, which can damage tissue.

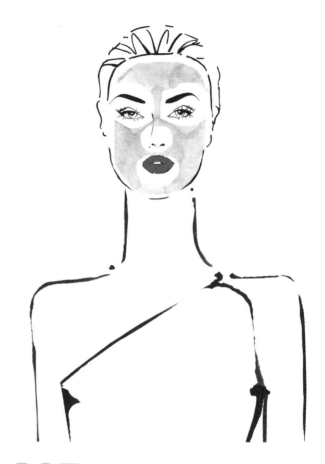

897 CLARIFY WITH CLAY

If you suffer from red, inflamed blemishes, use a clay-based mask or drying lotion to help draw out any impurities and reduce swelling. If the rest of your skin is dry, apply only to the affected area.

898 WASH WHITEHEADS AWAY

Keep whiteheads at bay on spot-prone skin by washing greasy areas with a mild cleanser containing benzoyl peroxide and glycolic acids, which in combination have been shown to reduce the severity of pimples.

899 STEM THE ERUPTION

Cystic acne has the potential to leave deep scars so spots should never be squeezed. For open pimples, apply an acne-drying gel or lotion and let it run its course. If you have frequent outbreaks including recurring spots and boils, consult a dermatologist. They will prescribe a specific course of action that neither your pharmacist nor your regular GP has the expertise to diagnose. Allowing the problem to linger means months without a solution.

900 WORK AWAY WHITEHEADS

If you suffer whiteheads, try applying a gel or cream containing salicylic acid to the pimple, a drying and toning agent that may help you to unplug the pores and prevent further outbreaks.

901 DON'T DRY IT OUT

You may think acne sufferers don't need moisturizer but never apply a blanket rule without considering your own skin. Many acne products contain drying ingredients that can leave skin red and irritated. Choose a good, light, hydrating moisturizer to help avoid tightness.

902 USE A SUNSCREEN

Sunscreen doesn't cause or "dry out" acne. In fact, some people find their acne worsens in the sun because the damaging effects actually encourage more oil production. At peak times, stay out of the sun and use a mineral (zinc oxide) sunblock rather than chemical blocks containing benzophenone and PABA.

903 MISS OUT THE MASK

If your skin suffers acne and breakouts, a mask may not be the best thing – even if it contains drying ingredients, it can actually clog up the skin. Instead use cleansers and toners to unblock pores and apply as little covering product as possible.

904 CHOOSE INGREDIENTS CAREFULLY

Products containing ingredients such as hyaluronic acid and glycerin help hold moisture in the skin without increasing oil production, so they're a great choice for oily or acne-prone skin.

905 CUT THE CLOG

Those with skin prone to acne and breakouts should never use heavy or oily products that can clog the skin, such as cocoa butter, mineral oil or cold cream. Instead look for light, non-greasy formulations.

906 PEROXIDE FOR PIMPLES

If you're prone to spotty breakouts, use a benzoyl peroxide solution on the affected area, which will dry out the oil and also has antibacterial properties, which can help prevent spots from appearing.

907 GO ANTI-BACTERIAL

There are two products on the market that help kill the bacteria that can contribute to acne infections – look for benzoyl peroxide and sodium sulfacetamide on labels.

908 GO NEUTRAL

Some brands of facial soap or facewash can have a very alkaline pH, which can dry out and irritate problem skin. Use a gentle, non-abrasive cleanser appropriate for your skin type instead.

909 TAKE THE ACID TEST

Face washes and cleansers containing salicylic acid are a good choice for acne because it helps clear away blocked pores and reduces redness and inflammation. Look, too, for cleansers containing emollients like lanolin to hold moisture in the skin without blocking.

910 APPLY IT ALL OVER

If you have problem skin on other areas of your body, use your acne products on them too, and follow the same routine.

911 DON'T USE A CLOTH

Avoid using a washcloth, sponge or muslin, which could lead to the spread of bacteria. Instead, wash your hands then use fingertips to gently rub cleanser into your face before rinsing with warm water.

open pores & blackheads

912 HEAT IT UP

If you must squeeze blackheads, apply a warm-to-hot flannel first to soften, then wrap a tissue around your fingers and gently squeeze. Never squeeze facial skin hard enough to leave an imprint.

913 TREAT SPOTS WITH FACIALS

Regular professionally administered facials can help prevent spots because they keep your pores cleaner than you can at home. Facial muscles are encouraged to relax and skin is kept hydrated and plump too.

914 PORES FOR THOUGHT

The best way to keep pores looking smaller and tighter is to keep them clean. Wash your face twice a day – morning and night – with a mild cleanser. If you have very large pores, use an astringent cleanser as well.

915 STEAM IT AWAY

It's almost impossible to prevent blackheads, but steam can help minimize them. Once a week, steam your face to soften the oils that clog the pores and follow with a deep-cleansing clay skin mask. Afterwards, rinse well with warm water to clear the skin.

916 UNPLUG BLACKHEADS

One of the most effective ways to rid yourself of blackheads without damaging or bruising the skin is with pore-cleaning strips (available over the counter from most pharmacies). Because the skin is not squeezed with this technique, it is not at risk from further infection.

917 STAY OUT OF THE SUN

Sun damage – both long-term and short-term – makes pores appear larger because UV rays break down collagen, making the tissues around your pores weaker and causing the epidermis to thicken. The effects can be permanent, so prevention is best.

pigmentation

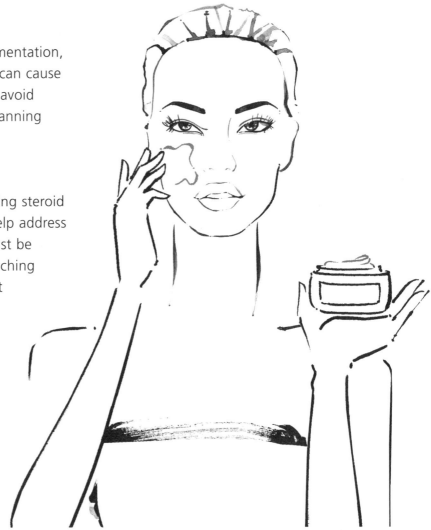

918 PIGMENT SKIN ALERT

If you suffer from irregular skin pigmentation, avoid bergamot essential oil as this can cause uneven skin colour to worsen. Also avoid exposure to the sun, sun lamps or tanning booths if using the oil.

919 AVOID BLEACH FOR VITILIGO

Repigmentation programmes involving steroid creams, UV light and surgery can help address the white patches of vitiligo but must be administered by a professional. Bleaching agents have side effects and are not the best option for dark skins.

920 BOTTLE THE MOTTLE

If you have mottled skin or patchy colouring, many heavy, penetrating moisturizers can help disguise and correct uneven pigmentation, giving the complexion a smoother, more even appearance. To prevent further problems, opt for one with built-in sunscreen.

921 HIDE BEHIND THE SCREEN

If you notice pigment patches on your cheeks or forehead, wear high-protection sunscreen at all times to minimize further damage and ensure your skin stays as even as possible.

922 PRESS THE CRESS

Cress has been shown to have beneficial effects in combating pigmentation, liver spots and age spots by helping the body regulate its melatonin levels. All types and colours of skin appear brighter and more even in tone.

923 KEEP IT SIMPLE

If you suffer from irregular pigmentation, keep your skincare routine simple. Avoid harsh sponges and exfoliating rubs – and don't use toner, which can exacerbate pigment differences.

924 GO ALGAL

Certain compounds in the red algae *Palmaria palmata* can help limit the transportation of pigment-containing melanosomes in the skin's deepest layers. This reduces the amount of pigment made, and consequently reduces areas of darker pigmentation.

broken veins

925 STAY COOL TO CURE CAPILLARIES

For the ultimate in smooth, blemish-free skin, try to stay cool. Overheating can cause damage to the fine capillaries in the cheeks and nose, which may contribute to and worsen any redness and blotchiness.

926 QUICK COVER UP

One of the best ways to reduce the visibility of broken veins is self-tanning lotion, which darkens the skin by a shade or two to reduce the contrast between skin and veins. If you're not sure about permanent colour, use a leg bronzer daily on affected areas.

927 GO SCLERO

One effective treatment for leg veins is sclerotherapy, where a solution is injected into individual veins to collapse them and force the blood to find another route, so reducing swelling and the visibility of veins and discomfort.

bruising & swelling

928 ASK FOR ARNICA

Arnica has long been known to help reduce swelling and bruising after damage to the skin because of the way it reduces the skin's inflammatory response to injury. Choose natural oils or creams to deliver a concentrated dose to reduce redness and puffiness on all skin areas.

929 BREW UP A CURE

For a home-made cure for bruises and swelling, boil up some leaves of Herb Robert (*Geranium robertianum*). While still warm, use as a poultice to lay over the affected area.

930 DO A DITTY

Dit Da Jow is a traditional Chinese remedy used for bruising. It contains substances such as myrrh, witch hazel, goldenseal, cinnamon, comfrey, arnica and ginseng, which help reduce both the pain and the appearance of the bruise.

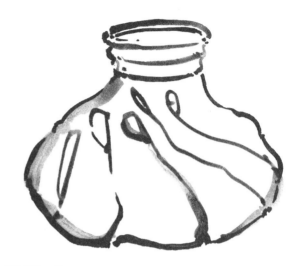

931 ICE IT

Did you know that the colour of bruises is caused by bleeding beneath the skin when small blood vessels are damaged? Applying a cold pack or ice pack immediately helps prevent bleeding from occurring, so reducing the appearance of the bruise.

932 GO LIGHT

Because of the blue and green tones beneath the skin it's best to choose a concealer or foundation a shade lighter than your skin tone to cover up a bruise. By the time it's applied, the bruise colour will tone it down.

933 ELEVATE

The best tip for reducing swelling is to harness the power of gravity by elevating the affected area above the heart and relaxing for 10 to 15 minutes.

cold sores

934 C THE DIFFERENCE

If you are prone to cold sores, take a daily supplement of vitamin C. A lack of the substance is thought to increase their frequency and longevity. Cold sores are likely to appear where skin is broken or damaged, so avoid extremes of environment such as hot and dry, windy, cold and very wet – and always protect your lips using a lip salve too.

935 ICE IT

At the onset of a cold sore, when you feel that telltale tinge, apply an ice cube wrapped in a plastic bag or piece of kitchen paper for two minutes, every 10 minutes for an hour. This will reduce the outbreak.

936 SAY NO TO CHOCLATE

It is thought that cold sores thrive on the amino acid arginine but are reduced by its partner, lysine. Redress your balance by avoiding chocolate, nuts, seeds, shellfish, grains and berries and fill up on dairy products, meat, avocados, apples, fish and soy. Or take a lysine supplement.

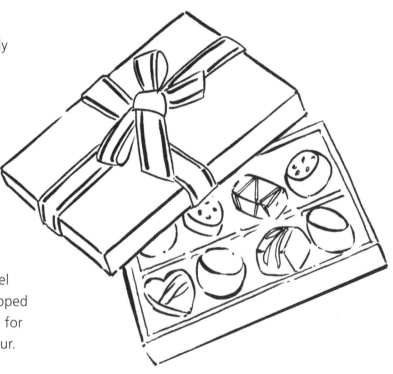

937 LEAVE IT ALONE

Cold sores are catching so they're best left alone. Apply minimal make-up and products to cover them, avoid exfoliating or using harsh products in their vicinity and wash hands thoroughly to avoid spreading.

938 DON'T SHARE

When you have a cold sore, avoid sharing towels, pillows, clothes, scarves and other fabrics to prevent spreading the virus to other people or elsewhere on your own body. Also, consult your doctor or pharmacist for advice on antiviral creams.

eczema

939 GET DIRTY

Mudpacks are a good choice for eczema as they contain high levels of nutrients as well as beneficial bacteria. Mix up a paste with water and mud, smear onto eczema and leave for 5–10 minutes. Be careful not to use on areas of cracked or chapped skin, though – it could introduce infection.

940 STAY COOL

Eczema symptoms can be exacerbated by extremes of temperature and respond particularly badly to overheating. Make sure you stay cool by seeking shade and choosing natural fabrics. Changing your laundry detergent may also help.

941 HIP TO BE ROSE

For dry skin, choose products containing extract of rosehip. This ingredient contains high levels of omega-3 and omega-6 oils, which are nourishing for the skin. It also acts as an anti-inflammatory to soothe problem areas.

942 DRIER THAN DUST

For skin tightness, cracking and flaking, choose a cream cleanser rather than a soap-based one and never use drying toners.

943 USE LESS ON ECZEMA

When it comes to covering sensitive skin conditions such as eczema, less is definitely more. Use too much powder or base and you risk highlighting the dryness and uneven texture of the skin.

944 RUB-A-DUB-DUB!

To reduce the severity of eczema, rub a whole nutmeg against a smooth stone, or grate with a very fine grater. Add water to the powder, mix to form a smooth paste and apply to the eczema. You could similarly use mustard powder, frankincense, turmeric or sandalwood.

945 DO A CLEOPATRA

If you suffer from eczema all over your body, try bathing in milk. Instead of filling a bath, which would be expensive and wasteful, use a bowl and give yourself a milky sponge bath. Leave for 10 minutes before showering off. Alternatively, add a cupful of milk powder to your usual soak.

946 GET GREASY

Oils are often a great choice for helping to reduce eczema symptoms as they stick around on the skin, so they carry on adding moisture for longer than lotions. For best results, use coconut oil, shea butter or cocoa butter in combination with glycerin or other skin-coating substances.

947 BLOW IT UP

The red, blistering itchy skin of eczema can be treated with a TriCeram cream, a non-steroid with a ceramide base that encourages the skin to repair itself. Balloon vine extract is an anti-inflammatory that also helps and is available in gel form.

948 GET ON YOUR SOAP BOX

Make your own anti-eczema soap by grating a large block of olive or vegetable soap into a bowl. Add a tablespoon of oatmeal, a handful of camomile flowers and a handful of rose petals, plus a few drops of rose and camomile essential oils. Heat gently and mix well, then leave to set in a mould lined with waxed paper.

under-eye bags & puffiness

948 SAY NO TO CAFFEINE

In the short term, caffeine might perk you up but that short-term alertness masks the long-term effects, which make you less likely to sleep well. It also causes mild dehydration, which can make dark circles appear worse.

950 APPLY CAUTION

Some skin-lightening creams, advertised for use in the under-eye area, may actually contain illegal compounds that can have negative effects on skin and health. Always seek advice from a qualified dermatologist before you use skin-lightening cream.

951 SAY OK FOR K

Vitamin K, when contained in skin treatment products, can help reduce the appearance of under-eye bags by boosting the skin's self-healing mechanism. Laser treatments can also help to do this, but many people are loath to risk lasers so near their eyes.

952 FILL IT IN

If your under-eye bags are due to broken capillaries or to fat loss because of ageing, or if the collagen and elastin in your skin breaks down due to ageing, a dermatologist may advise injectable fillers. Performed correctly, these can help smooth out the skin and make it appear plumper and more even in tone.

953 SLEEP IT OFF

The single most effective thing you can do to reduce under-eye bags is to get enough sleep. Not only does this help to keep the inside of the eyes bright, so minimizing the appearances of dark circles, but it also allows the skin to repair damage and rebalance the melanin that causes colour changes.

954 VISIT THE ROSE GARDEN

Rosewater, either over-the-counter or made yourself by steeping crushed rose petals in water overnight, is a great way to reduce baggy eyes as it helps moisturize and calm swelling at the same time. Apply using a warm or cold towel, depending on which you find more relaxing.

955 COOL IT

Using cold compresses can be a great way to reduce puffy eyes because it prevents so much blood flowing to the skin and calms redness. Use chilled moist teabags, slices of cucumber, a cold pack of peas (wrap in a tea towel) or a gel eye mask and relax for 10 minutes.

956 SPLASH IT AWAY

To reduce swelling and puffiness, splash cold water on your face in the morning to "wake up" your facial circulation. Splash several times to keep water on your face for several minutes rather than splashing just once, as this will be more effective.

psoriasis

957 GET AN EXTREME CURE

The drug methotrexate can halt the damaging effects of psoriasis, but it's hard to target just at the skin as it tends to have further reaching effects on the body than intended and is therefore only used in the most extreme cases.

958 SWILL A SARSAPARILLA

Sarsaparilla is a herb known to bind to toxins in the body and thus helps reduce the effects of psoriasis. Or try oregano, another powerful detoxifying agent. The herb milk thistle helps support the liver for the same purifying effect and also helps clear up problems.

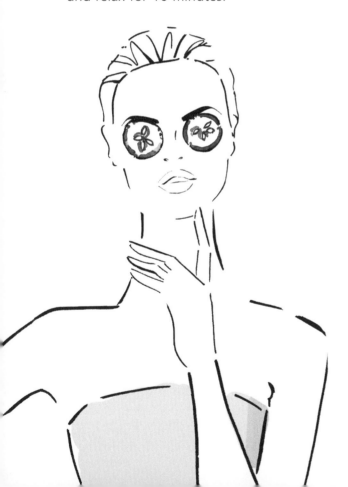

959 DIVE FOR DITHRANOL

Traditionally treated with coal tar and emollients, new creams containing vitamins D3 and A have proved beneficial. Dithranol, from the South American tree *Vataireopsis araroba*, has been proven to kill off the rapidly reproducing cells at the root of the problem. It can cause skin reactions, however, so avoid prolonged use and sensitive skin areas.

960 CHILL OUT

Psoriasis is due to a build up of skin cells that have grown and divided too quickly, causing skin growth many hundreds of times faster than normal. Scientists don't have the definitive answer but it is known to be linked to stress so if you are a sufferer, adding some counselling or relaxation therapy to your life could be beneficial.

961 SEARCH FOR SULPHUR

If you suffer any sort of inflammatory skin condition, including psoriasis, consider taking an MSM (sulphur) supplement. You can also increase sulphur-containing foods such as eggs, onions and garlic in your diet.

962 GET SOME UV THERAPY

Ultraviolet light therapy is a very useful treatment for most people with psoriasis, but because of the damaging effects of UV rays on the skin, it tends to be used in only small bursts. Get your own healing dose by making sure you spend at least half an hour in the sun, where possible, each day.

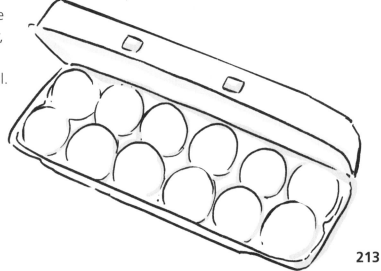

963 DON'T BE BITTER

Psoriasis is also linked to a sluggish digestive system. If you suffer from this or any other inflammatory skin condition, a herbal mixture called Swedish bitters can help to stimulate digestion, or choose Bromelain, derived from pineapple, which contains digestive enzymes.

964 WHIP SOME CREAM

Cortisone creams, although useful for reducing swelling, can also make skin thinner over time and in the long term, may exacerbate the problems. Look for milder natural alternatives such as glycyrrhetinic acid, which is derived from licorice, and camomile creams.

965 GET IN THE QUERCETIN

Quercetin is a plant bioflavonoid with powerful antioxidant properties that can help soothe inflammation. Taken alongside vitamins A and zinc, it's a great choice for inflammatory conditions such as psoriasis. Look for a supplement containing around 400 mg.

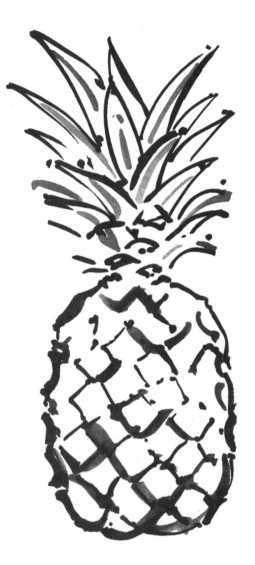

966 GET DEAD AHEAD

The Dead Sea has long been cited as the perfect holiday destination for those with psoriasis – the combination of bright sunlight and salty water helps calm and nurture skin. Create your own Dead Sea experience by filling a warm tub with a couple of handfuls of Epsom salts and a handful of salt, then soaking for 20 minutes.

967 BE A VEGGIE

People with psoriasis often find their condition is improved if they cut down dramatically on animal fats from red meat and dairy, which can cause inflammation in the body and worsen the condition. Cut these out of your diet for a few days to see if there is any improvement and reintroduce slowly.

968 BALANCE YOUR BODY

People with psoriasis often have reduced levels of protein and folic acid because their skin uses up so much as it grows (don't forget, the symptoms are caused by skin overgrowth). If you have this condition, make sure you get adequate proteins and B vitamins.

969 GET SEEDY

Seeds contain great fats and oils to help reduce inflammation and in turn reduce the effects of psoriasis, but many people don't like the taste of them. Invest in a coffee grinder and grind pumpkin, sunflower, safflower and hemp seeds together, then use as a sprinkle on cereals, salads and cooked food to get your health boost daily.

allergic reactions & rashes

970 BE AN ICE MAIDEN

Ice is useful for helping to calm allergic reactions as it can constrict blood flow to the area it is in contact with, so reducing swelling and itching. For skin reactions, apply directly inside a clean cloth or plastic bag. Alternatively, wet a cloth with cold milk and lie it directly on the affected area for five to 10 minutes for relief from skin allergies and itching, especially hives.

971 BATHE IT AWAY

For skin allergies, pour half a cup of baking soda into your bath and soak for around 20 minutes. This helps reduce redness, swelling and itching anywhere on the skin. For hard-to-soak areas, such as the face, soak a flannel in the mixture and apply to the area for several minutes, then rinse and pat dry.

972 GET SOME BALANCE

Some rashes are due to pH changes in the skin – regulate yours by dabbing on apple cider vinegar mixed with equal parts of lemon juice, then smear over some honey to help seal in the healing effects. After five to 10 minutes rinse off; apply a natural moisturizing oil, such as olive or almond.

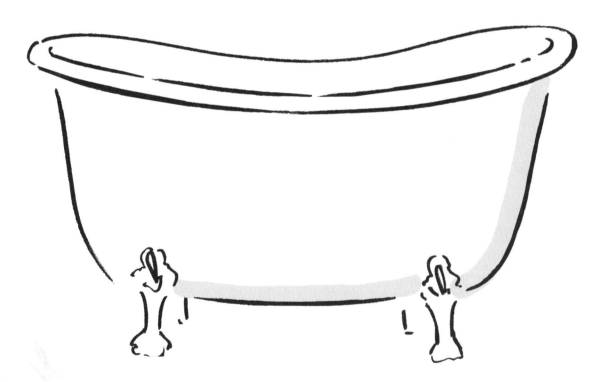

973 GET A POT

Potassium is essential for healthy skin, and if you suffer from bouts of dermatitis, you could be deficient in the mineral. Get yours from avocados, apricots, bananas, beans, parsley, peaches, wheatgerm, carrots, dried fruits and soybeans. Alternatively, take a skin health supplement.

974 GO ON A WITCH HUNT

Witch hazel can help heal eczema and dermatitis if used on sore skin as soon as it starts to develop. Use the essential oil mixed with olive or almond oil so your skin is moisturized too, and apply three to five times a day as required.

975 BE A BASIL BATHER

To help relieve skin allergies, try washing the affected area in basil tea. Simply steep fresh basil leaves in hot water, cool, then strain and use as a rinse as often as needed. If your skin is red and itchy, add some cooling witch hazel or aloe vera as well.

976 FACIAL HARMONY

To improve red, itchy or allergic skin, visit a salon for a specific ultra-sensitive skin treatment. Plant-based products such as arnica and cypress nut can reduce swelling and redness.

977 SENSE YOUR SENSITIVITY

If your skin is reactive, try to find out the triggers, whether environmental, nutritional or from using certain skincare products. Bolster your skin's barrier with a moisturizer for sensitive skin and protect it from extremes of weather. Dehydrated skin is more susceptible to infections, immune disorders and sun damage.

978 AVOID THE PRICKLE

Prickly heat is a rash that develops when the sweat glands over-react to heat and humidity, causing red, itchy bumps to appear all over the skin. If you are prone to sweating, choose man-made fibres to help your skin cool naturally.

979 CALM WITH CAMOMILE

To soothe inflamed skin, dip a camomile teabag in warm water and hold the teabag onto the skin for a few minutes. Pat dry, reheat and repeat as needed.

980 CALL ON CALAMINE

Calamine lotion is a good choice for soothing angry skin as dries it out gently, avoiding side effects. Use as often as required to give relief.

981 TIP ON THE TEA TREE

Tea tree oil helps heal dermatitis where the skin has broken, and it also prevents infection from developing. If your skin is very sore or weeping, dilute the oil with a light vegetable oil.

982 DO SOME BLUE SKY THINKING

Blueberries and blueberry leaves contain high levels of antioxidants that can help reduce swelling and boost skin healing. Blend some blueberries and apply directly to skin as a mask; leave for 10 minutes before rinsing off.

freckles, moles & birthmarks

983 BE AWARE

The only moles that are really dangerous are those that look different from other existing moles or that appear after the age of 25. Any mole that bleeds, oozes, itches or changes size or colour should be professionally checked as soon as possible.

984 MAKE A PACT

If a malignant melanoma is caught early on, there's a good chance of recovery, so it's vital to check your skin regularly. Make a pact with a friend, partner or relative to check each other's moles once a month for any changes.

985 CHECK ALL OVER

Melanomas start from moles so it's a good idea to look out for changes, particularly bleeding, changing shape, itching, colour or sensation. Remember to check hard-to-see areas, such as your back, joints and scalp, and seek professional advice if you notice any changes.

986 KNOW YOUR ALPHABET

Follow the ABCDE of mole checking: Asymmetry (do the sides match?); Border (is it fractured or smooth?); Colour (is it uniform and free from flecks of black, brown, blue, white or red?); Diameter (is it wider than a pencil eraser?); and Evolution (is it changing?). If the answer to any of these is yes, seek immediate medical advice.

warts, verrucas & other infections

987 GET IN THE HOUSE

A great cure for warts and verrucas is the house leek, or *Sempervivum*, which is high in supermalate of calcium. Take a fleshy leaf, cut it in half lengthways to expose the inner flesh and juice, then take one half of the leaf to squeeze juice directly onto the wart; use a plaster to stick the other exposed side onto the skin. Change every 12 or 24 hours and continue until the wart disappears.

988 A SLIVER OF SILVER

Colloidal silver, painted on top of the wart, has been shown to be effective against viruses of all sorts. Ask your doctor for advice on where to find and how to use.

989 TAKE SOME TEA

Warts are caused by a virus so dabbing them with aromatherapy oils with anti-viral properties might help reduce them. Onion oil, garlic oil and tea tree oil are all good choices, or you could rub a raw garlic clove or slice of onion onto the wart instead.

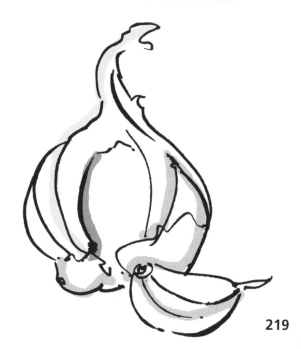

980 COVER IT UP

Some scientists believe the presence of warts and verrucas on the skin is a sign that the body's immune system doesn't recognize the virus as an impostor. They suggest keeping the wart constantly covered with a plaster to encourage the immune system to engage in that area of skin and thus "discover" the problem and get rid of it.

981 PICK A PINEAPPLE

Pineapples are rich in digestive enzymes, which some believe can help dissolve warts and verrucas. Soak a piece of cotton wool, muslin or sterile dressing in pineapple juice and apply directly to the area, preferably taping it on overnight. Saliva contains some similar enzymes, so could be used as an alternative.

982 SPEND A PENNY

Soak a copper penny in vinegar until the mixture turns green and then bathe your wart or verruca in the mixture every night before bed. The copper ions are thought to help reduce wart growth.

983 RUB IT OUT

The leaves of the rubber plant (*Hevea brasiliensis*) can be used to get rid of warts and verrucas. Break a leaf from the plant and paint the white oozing liquid onto the affected area. Repeat five to six times a day until the wart or verruca disappears.

984 FLIP AND FLOP

To avoid catching a verruca, footwear should always be worn in public places and feet should be kept clean, dry and away from moist floors, like changing rooms and public showers. If you swim regularly or use changing rooms where the floor is likely to be wet, invest in a pair of flip flops.

985 JUICE UP AN APPLE

Once a day, try soaking your wart or verruca in the juice of a sour apple, which is high in magnesium. Choose a variety that is sour rather than sweet – look for Bramley cooking apples, Cox and Granny Smith, which all have less sugar than sweeter varieties.

996 JUICE A CURE

The juice or milk of several different plants, when applied to a wart or verruca once or twice a day and covered by a bandage, is believed to help rid the body of the virus that causes them. Try cabbage, green fig, dandelion and chickweed.

997 PLAY THE WAITING GAME

Most experts believe the best way to get rid of warts and verrucas is to wait until they go. It's rare to have one for more than two years and so long as they don't get infected (avoid picking or knocking them), they should leave no scar.

athlete's foot

998 BE SUNNY

Where possible, expose your feet to sunlight for at least an hour every day. Natural sunlight kills the fungus that causes athlete's foot, so getting out and about is a great natural remedy.

999 CRUSH SOME GARLIC

Crush a garlic clove and apply to the area affected with athlete's foot. Leave for 30 minutes before rinsing off with warm water. Do this once a day to help beat athlete's foot. If the garlic should burn your skin, remove and rinse immediately.

1000 GO GINGER

Ginger has anti-fungal properties, so it's a great treatment for athlete's foot. Infuse some ginger root in hot water, cool and then use as a foot-soak for 15 minutes twice a day. Tea tree oil, applied directly to the affected area two or three times a day, can also help.

1001 GET TOUCHY-FEELY

Using grapefruit seed oil to massage feet twice daily can help remove athlete's foot as the extract is an anti-fungal. Make up your own foot lotion using grapefruit seed extract, a carrier oil such as almond and a few drops of tea tree oil.

INDEX

Author's Acknowledgements

Thanks as usual to everyone who's helped me with the vast amount of information needed for writing this book: Clare Rogers at the Treatment Rooms in Brighton, simply the best day spa in my world!; Pauline Floyd, always a source of obscure plant knowledge; Mel Amin, Nicola Cracknell, Luisa Collett, Jo Philpot and Jules Rogers – just for understanding! Kevin, Freddie and Joe for reminding me constantly how important laughter is. And finally to my beloved Grandma, May Curson, for still having fabulous skin at the age of 101 … Every day, in every way, a little better!